PSYCHOSOCIAL FAMILY INTERVENTIONS IN CHRONIC PEDIATRIC ILLNESS

THE DOWNSTATE SERIES OF
RESEARCH IN PSYCHIATRY AND PSYCHOLOGY

A Continuation Order Plan is available for this series. A continuation order will bring delivery of each new volume immediately upon publication. Volumes are billed only upon actual shipment. For further information please contact the publisher.

Psychosocial Family Interventions in Chronic Pediatric Illness

Edited by

ADOLPH E. CHRIST

and

KALMAN FLOMENHAFT

Downstate Medical Center Brooklyn, New York

PLENUM PRESS · NEW YORK AND LONDON

Library of Congress Cataloging in Publication Data

Symposium on Family Dynamics, Family Therapy and Pediatric Medical Illness (1980: Downstate
  Medical Center, N.Y.)
  Psychosocial family interventions in chronic pediatric illness.

  (Downstate series of research in psychiatry and psychology; v. 3)
  "Proceedings of a Symposium on Family Dynamics, Family Therapy and Pediatric Medical Illness, held December 12 – 13, 1980, at Downstate Medical Center, Brooklyn, New York."
  Bibliography: p.
  Includes index.
  1. Chronic diseases in children—Psychological aspects—Congresses. 2. Chronically ill
children—Family relationships—Congresses. 3. Family psychotherapy—Congresses. I. Christ,
Adolph E. II. Flomenhaft, Kalman. III. Title. IV. Series. [DNLM: 1. Chronic disease—In infancy and
childhood—Congresses. 2. Chronic disease—Psychology—Congresses. 3. Family
therapy—Congresses. 4. Parent – child relations—Congresses. W1 D0945 v. 4/WS 200 S9875p 1980]
RJ380.S95 1980   155.9′16   82-5309
ISBN 978-1-4684-4249-6   ISBN 978-1-4684-4247-2 (eBook)   AACR2
DOI 10.1007/978-1-4684-4247-2

Proceedings of a Symposium on Family Dynamics, Family Therapy
and Pediatric Medical Illness, held December 12 – 13, 1980, at
Downstate Medical Center, Brooklyn, New York

© 1982 Plenum Press, New York
Softcover reprint of the hardcover 1st edition 1982
A Division of Plenum Publishing Corporation
233 Spring Street, New York, N.Y. 10013

FOREWORD

The symposium "Family Dynamics, Family Therapy, and Pediatric Medical Illness," held at Downstate Medical Center on December 12 and 13, 1980, considered the impact of life-threatening illness in children and adolescents on intrafamilial dynamics. A group of experts addressed the practical and theoretical psychological and social issues facing pediatric patients and their families when confronting chronic and severe childhood illnesses including brain damage, cancer, hemophilia, juvenile diabetes, and heart disease.

The presentations and group discussions clearly revealed the complexity of physical and psychological problems posed by the seriously ill child with chronic disease for both the health care provider and the family. The conference proceedings confirm that quality care and treatment for the ill child requires the participation of a variety of health care disciplines representing diverse fields of knowledge. Pediatricians, family practitioners, child psychiatrists, nurses, social workers, psychologists, nutritionists and others all have important collaborative roles to play.

The symposium participants wrestled with some of the basic developmental and clinical questions: How is the ongoing development of a family altered as a result of chronic incapacitating illness in a child member? How can principles of intensive family and individual psychotherapy be applied during the medical treatment of life-threatening illness? What are the psychological stress points during the course of a chronic medical illness? These are but a few of the issues addressed in this publication.

I am convinced that the future of the mental health field must include substantially better integration of medical and psychiatric perspectives. This volume helps to move us in this direction.

Donald Scherl, M.D.
President
Downstate Medical Center

v

PREFACE

Family theory is increasing our understanding and treatment
of pediatric medical illness. There is a developing body of
knowledge on the effects of a child's illness on the family, the
way a child's illness may be an outcome of certain aspects of
family life and stress, the role of the family and the health care
team in enhancing compliance to the medical regimen of the patient,
and the prevention of maladaptation in the siblings of the seriously
ill child.

These issues were addressed in the symposium "Family Dynamics,
Family Therapy and Pediatric Medical Illness" conducted in December,
1980 at Downstate Medical Center. During this meeting, a group
of experts dealt with the practical and theoretical issues affecting children and adolescents who are faced with chronic and life
threatening illnesses including cancer, brain damage, hemophilia,
juvenile diabetes, and heart disease.

The contributors revealed an extraordinary sensitivity
to the emotional and physical turmoil of parents who have seriously
ill children. The presentations were marked by conceptual clarity
and clinical wisdom for the complex and perplexing psychological,
family, and social issues. The discussion periods and exchanges
between the presenters and symposium attendees were vital and
engrossing. Enough questions and issues were raised to warrant
a future symposium.

The success of the symposium was made possible by a number
of people: Mrs. Beverley DeSouza for making order out of the many
details of conducting a symposium and preparing this volume;
Mrs. Libby Cohen in arranging the symposium; Mr. Martin Nathanson
for his audio-visual services, and, finally, Mrs. Caroline
Apolito for typing the final manuscript.

Above all, the editors are thankful to the Elizabeth Berliss Saenger, M.D. Memorial Fund for sponsoring the symposium and to Downstate Medical Center and the Department of Psychiatry for their support.

Adolph E. Christ, M.D.

Kalman Flomenhaft, Ph.D.

CONTENTS

THE CHALLENGE OF PEDIATRIC MEDICAL ILLNESS TO FAMILY THEORY AND FAMILY THERAPY

Adolph E. Christ, M.D.

Downstate Medical Center-Kings County Hospital

Brooklyn, New York

What are the challenges that medical illness brings to the mental health profession? A number will emerge in the chapters that follow. The one I would like to emphasize is: Can we reorient our perspective and deal with those problems in the family with a medically ill child that might require us to alter our basic psychiatric perspectives, theories, and therapies, rather than, as we have in the past, with the applications of our theories and expertise to the physically ill child and his family?

Let me exemplify this point. Our early involvement with medical illness, especially with the "psychosomatic diseases," was a straightforward application of whatever psychiatric theory and practice was available and of interest at the time. Franz Alexander's (1961) search for the etiologic conflict for specific symptoms led him to emphasize, for example, that conflicts with aggression could manifest themselves as headaches, as hypertension, or as rheumatoid arthritis. This is clearly an application of the principles that were so useful to S. Freud (1923) in his understanding of the physical symptoms of the hysteric. Flanders Dunbar (1943) took another important parameter of psychiatric theory and looked not for the specific etiologic conflicts, but rather at the personality types that would predictably develop one rather than another syndrome. Another example of our interest in using psychiatric insights in understanding and treating the physically ill population comes closer to the topic of this book. The parent as etiologic in the causation of psychiatric illness in the child is exemplified in the early thinking about the family--Fromm-Reichsman's (1948) schizophrenogenic mother and Gregory Bateson's (1958) double-bind theory depicting the role of the parent in the etiology of schizo-

phrenic illness find parallel expression in the removal of the
asthmatic child from the family, in the use of "parentectomy" as a
therapeutic tool (1963). Even closer to our conference, and to those
of us interested in family therapy, are the findings of Minuchin
et al. (1975) of the effectiveness of the use of structural family
therapy techniques with severe diabetic and asthmatic children.
Here again, we see an example of the application of psychiatric
principles and techniques to physical illness.

Most of us have arrived at an acceptance of the usefulness of
von Bertalanffy's (1968) systems theory, with the invaluable concepts
of multidimensionality and equifinality. No longer are we tied to
a simple zero order correlation--one cause one effect paradigm.
Even the statistical tool of Multiple Regression/Correlation Analysis
(1975) can now, through the square of the correlations and the semi-
partial correlations give us a percentage of the variance that can
be accounted for by each of a number of variables. We could now
theoretically ask, for example, how much of the variance in a
population of ill people can be accounted for by conflict, by personality type, by parental etiologic causation of the illness,
and by family malstructure. If each of these perspectives were
associated with an effective therapy whose outcome we could measure,
we could even ask, as we might predict from the principle of equifinality, how much of the variance in the improvement of patients
with a specific illness could be accounted for by each of these
therapies?

We have come a long way. However, I am left a bit uneasy by
this pre-Copernican perspective. Should we perhaps also ask what
may there be in physical illness and its effect on the child and
his family that may alter our predominant psychiatric perspective,
or as Freud emphasized, "Weltanschauung?" Humanity gained a great
deal from the pre-Copernican perspective of earth as the center of
the universe, but also from the humbling perspective of our solar
system as but a speck in an insignificant spiral of our galaxy, and
our galaxy as but one of countless others.

We chose topics that appear in the rest of this book, such
as genetic illness, neurologic illness, cancer, heart disease, to
see where our current thinking about the medically ill child and
his family can bring us. There is one important point that is made
by a number of the authors. Although clearly not as narcissism
injuring as the Copernican revolution, we are faced with one factor
that we need to address: To think about coping and adapting to these
illnesses, another currently important mental health concept, is not
the whole story in thinking about the families of the medically ill
child. Rather, as you will read, the presence of these illnesses
in a child, in a sibling, in a parent, will significantly and
profoundly alter the whole course of the lives of the individuals
and of the family. The challenge of experiences with medical illness

is: What can we offer to the family, to the siblings, whose life is inevitably altered by such a profound experience? Can we prevent the serious destructive consequences for some of the families, even unto the next generation, of catastrophic events such as the severe lifelong or mortal illness of one of the members?

As a profession, we are working on defining the "normal" or "expected" sequence of development in individuals and in families. Although last year's symposium dealt with the teaching of family therapy, most presenters focused on some aspects of this area of emerging family theory. For example, Saul Brown (1980) outlined six phases in the developmental cycle of families; Charles Malone (1980) stressed the complementary links between dyanmic child psychiatry and family therapy, highlighting the place of dynamic developmental concepts in relation to the core clinical issues in family therapy; Grunebaum and Chasin (1980) highlighted the importance of the historical perspective in looking at families; Wells Goodrich (1980) spoke of family developmental stage disturbance as one of three family system intervention organizers. Clearly, family development is at the cutting edge of the development of family theory.

Medical illness faces us with a different perspective on family development. I find that the more catastrophic medical illness experiences result in an unalterable new course of family development consequent to that experience. Within the new course, there may be more or less adaptive responses by the family. Can it be that catastrophic medical illness challenges us to understand not one, but perhaps a series of "normal" and "abnormal" developmental sequences for families? That piece of family theory would be invaluable to the mental health clinician who is dealing with a family during the acute crisis. Perhaps only then could we truly prevent the abnormal development of family members within the context of the altered or alternative developmental sequence.

This is not totally virgin territory. Efforts to understand the consequences of the concentration camp experience, to understand the effects of calamities such as the Three Mile Harbor Nuclear accident and the much earlier Coconut Grove (Lindemann, 1976) fire, and Hiroshima (Lifton, 1976) atom bomb point to a recognition that events can have effects beyond the expected duration of the catastrophy. We need to focus on understanding the totally altered life sequences, even unto the next generation, that are attendant upon traumatic, catastrophic, life events.

REFERENCES

Alexander, F. The Psychosomatic Approach in Medical Therapy (1954). In F. Alexander (Ed.) The Scope of Psychoanalysis 1921-1961. New York: Basic Books, 1961.

Bateson, G., Jackson, D., Haley, J. and Weakland, J. Toward a
    Theory of Schizophrenia. Behavioral Science, 1:251-264, 1958.
Bertalanffy, L. V. General Systems Theory--A Critical Review.
    In W. Buckley (Ed.) Modern Systems Research for the Behavioral
    Scientist, Chicago: Aldine, 1968.
Brown, S. L. Comprehension of the Developmental Cycle of Families
    in the Training of Child Psychiatry Clinicians. In
    K. Flomenhaft and A. E. Christ (Eds.) The Challenge of,Family
    Therapy: A Dialogue for Child Psychiatric Educators. New York:
    Plenum, 1980.
Cohen, J. and Cohen, P. Applied Multiple Regression/Correlation
    Analysis for the Behavioral Sciences. New York: Wiley, 1975.
Dunbar, H. F. Psychosomatic Diagnosis. New York: Hoeber, 1943.
Flomenhaft, K. and Christ, A. E. (Eds.) The Challenge of Family
    Therapy: A Dialogue for Child Psychiatric Educators, New York:
    Plenum, 1980.
Freud, S. (1905) Fragment of an Analysis of a Case of Hysteria.
    Collected Papers, Vol. III, 13-146, 1923.
Fromm-Reichmann, F. Notes on the Development of Treatment of
    Schizophrenics by Psychoanalytic Psychotherapy. Psychiatry,
    11:263-273, 1948.
Goodrich, W. Introduction of Family Therapy into Child Psychiatry
    Training: Two Styles of Change. In K. Flomenhaft and A. E.
    Christ (Eds.) The Challenge of Family Therapy: A Dialogue for
    Child Psychiatric Educators, New York: Plenum, 1980.
Grunebaum, H. and Chasin, R. Thinking Like a Family Therapist. In
    K. Flomenhaft and A. E. Christ (Eds.) The Challenge of Family
    Therapy: A Dialogue for Child Psychiatric Educators. New York:
    Plenum, 1980.
Lifton, R. L. Psychological Effects of the Atomic Bomb in Hiroshima:
    The Theme of Death. In R. Fulton (Ed.) Death and Identity,
    London: Prentice-Hall, 1976.
Lindemann, E. Symptomatology and Management of Acute Grief. In
    R. Fulton (Ed.) Death and Identity, London: Prentice-Hall, 1976.
Malone, C. A. Family Therapy and Child Psychiatric Training: Issues,
    Problems, and Strategies. In K. Flomenhaft and A. E. Christ
    (Eds.) The Challenge of Family Therapy: A Dialogue for Child
    Psychiatric Educators. New York: Plenum, 1980.
Minuchin, S., Baker, L., Rosman, B. L. A Conceptual Model of
    Psychosomatic Illness in Children. Archives of General
    Psychiatry, 32:1021-1038, 1975.
Peshkin, M. Diagnosis of Asthma in Children: Past and Present.
    In H. I. Schneer (Ed.) The Asthmatic Child: Approach to
    Problems and Treatment. New York: Harper and Row, 1963.

THE FAMILY AND MEDICAL ILLNESS

Kalman Flomenhaft, Ph.D.

Downstate Medical Center-Kings County Hospital

Brooklyn, New York

Society's current interest in the family stems from a variety
of forces including political, economic, and social. No doubt, the
rise of many alternative family styles and the decline of the traditional family structure of father as breadwinner, mother as full-time
homemaker, and two-plus children generates this interest. The
traditional family, even the entire concept of the family, has been
assaulted and battered, and its extinction, altogether, has been
predicted (Cooper, 1971). Nevertheless, there appears to be more
and more concern to assist and support the family, whatever the
structure, to meet the increasing challenges and responsibilities
being placed on it.

The mental health professions have been focusing increasingly
on the family. Family systems theory and therapy are an increasing
part of the theoretical and clinical repertoire of many practicing
mental health professionals, including psychiatrists, social workers,
nurses, and psychologists. Until fairly recently, psychiatric
diagnostic procedures and treatment methods focused primarily on
the identified patient. The patient's family was viewed as a
necessary ally in problem management, but not as having made a significant contribution to the problem. Currently, a marked shift in
emphasis has taken place. The family is now conceptualized as both
the etiology of and means by which many psychiatric and emotional
problems can be understood and treated (Bloch, 1974).

FAMILY THEORY AND PHYSICAL ILLNESS

Family systems theory, however, has given little consideration
to physical illness and disease. An early review of the psychosomatic literature by Grolnick (1972) found little work "really

concerned with the relationships of interactional patterns and physical illness." Weakland's (1977) more recent analysis of the psychosomatic medicine literature determined the emphasis was largely "an individualistic one, or at most a mother-child orientation to psychological factors in disease." It appears, therefore, that we have not responded to the challenge posed by Meissner (1966) over 15 years ago when he wrote:

> The awareness has grown in recent years that human disease, in addition to a pathology, also has an ecology. The understanding of disease, then, must comprehend the pertinent aspect of that ecology if it is to be at all meaningful. The patient's emotional involvement in the family system constitutes a major aspect of that ecology which we can no longer afford to ignore.

This symposium is timely and pioneering to consider the biological, psychological, and social context of individuals who are faced with serious and life-threatening illness. This gathering also reflects the increasing application of family systems theory to physical problems. The increasing interest in family systems theory cannot be solely attributed to its capacity to increase our understanding of illness, to its potential utility, or to the handful of theorists and clinicians who advocate it zealously. For a theory to be generally accepted, the preceding is not enough, because, in addition, there must be the right kind of economic, societal and political climate to enhance the theory's acceptance.

CHANGING HEALTH CARE PATTERNS

What is that climate? Clearly, our society is increasingly examining the interaction of the cost, quality, effectiveness, and humaneness of health care. The American Medical Association (1978) highlights the issue of cost in a recently released report:

> After years of emphasizing access to and quality of care, society is calling to question the cost of delivering this care. After years of consumers wanting unlimited care, government promoting growth in the production of both providers and facilities and physicians providing service based solely on quality, it is necessary to instill alternative behavior patterns for everyone.

Additionally, there is dawning realization and reluctant acceptance of the limits and uncertainty of medicine (Powles, 1979; Knowles, 1979). Individuals are taking more responsibility for their health, while drawing upon the strength and resources of their own natural support network (Gartner and Riessman, 1977). The development of alternative patterns and forms of health care--the feminist health movement, holistic health care, midwifery, home deliveries, home care--are partly a result of this examination (Ruzek, 1978; Sobel, 1979). Significant pressure for new directions in medicine has also come from within the profession. Some of these developments focus on new approaches to patient care. The notions of "primary care" and "comprehensive care" reflect the inclusion of more patient oriented factors. Mauksch (1974) notes that the emergence of the specialty of Family Medicine is symptomatic of a complex sense of discomfort within the health profession and by the public at large regarding the depersonalization and episodal discontinuity associated with the scientific advances of clinical medicine...an almost cyclical rediscovery of the human, social, and cultural aspects of health and illness.

REMEMBRANCE OF THINGS PAST

The developing family focus of health care makes me recall an aspect of my early life which was spent in Brooklyn. As a child, I remember my family's medical needs being attended to by one physician, a kindly gentleman with glasses, moustache, and ruffled hair, who always wore a fedora. This man was surgeon, family practitioner, obstetrician, gynecologist, orthopedist, psychiatrist, nurse, social worker, psychologist, and finally, his own receptionist and account-ant. He had delivered me; performed an appendectomy on my older brother; placed innumerable casts on my middle brother who was always breaking legs, arms, and ankles; performed a tonsillectomy on me in his office, and a hernia operation on my mother; treated my father for a variety of stomach ailments; and above all, he was a mediator and therapist for many of our family conflicts.

I cannot remember any member of my family being referred to a specialist, no matter the situation, the symptom, or the physical illness. Currently, a similar family raising three children would most likely have been referred to a variety of health care pro-fessionals. My family's contacts with him took place equally in his office and in our home. Whenever he came to our home to check on one member, invariably he would deal with everybody else's physical and emotional complaints. Intuitively, without having had a family therapy training program, he understood quite well my family's dynamics. He knew well how to walk a tightrope between my mother's persistent complaints and my father's absolute denial that anything was wrong. He grasped the emotional significance of many of the children's illnesses in terms of the family's dynamics and treated them accordingly. In many respects, he was the sixth member of our family. Just knowing that he was available in times of pain and illness was sufficient to tide us over a stressful period.

The quality of relationship my family of origin had with this physician has stayed with me throughout the years. I have tried to

recapture it for my own family, but without success. Our current
delivery and organization of medical care and the fact that I and
my family have lived in different parts of the country have made it
impossible to replicate this doctor-family-patient relationship. No
doubt, the greater sophistication of health care, with no one
professional trained and equipped to diagnose and treat the range
and variety of physical and emotional problems, work against the
development of this kind of relationship. True enough! But have
we lost something in the process? Does this something have any
relevance to the purpose of this symposium?

THE FAMILY AND THE HOSPITAL

     John Bell (1969, 1975) conducted a survey of medical and
psychiatric hospitals throughout the world for the World Health
Organization. What he found is of significance for this conference.
In many parts of the world, notably the less developed, the family
is involved much more in the treatment of the physically and psychiatrically ill individual. When hospitalizing an individual, the
entire family accompanies the patient to the hospital. In the
hospital, family members feed and care for the patient, allowing
hospital personnel to perform only those functions for the patient
that the family members are unable to do. In some instances, whole
communities become hospitals. The family is not the guest of the
hospital but develops a viable role as a legitimate health care
provider. Evidence suggests that the presence of family members in
patient care exerts a positive influence on patient health (Bell,
1975).

     Contrasting this practice to ours in the western world,
McWhinney (1975) notes, "The hospital tends by its very nature to
separate the disease from the man, and the man from his environment."
The emphasis of hospitalization is on restoration of illness-deter-
mined losses, rather than on the social, physical and environmental
totality of the patient. The medical staff tends to regard consideration of the family context as optional rather than integral. In
many instances, though, staffs have actively engaged families in
hospital pediatric care and mothers have been allowed to stay overnight with an ill child. Nowadays, fathers have more opportunity to
participate in the birth and delivery of their children. However,
in examining hospital programs, "no effective integration of the
patient-family unit into the hospital has been achieved, and too
often, staff assume an adversary position toward the family....little
importance is given to keeping alive family relationships (Shapiro,
1980)." The family role in health care, therefore, usually becomes
minimal and observational rather than major and participatory.
Transfer of caring skills to family members is either nonexistent or
incomplete.

SIGNIFICANCE OF CHRONIC DISEASE

Why am I stressing the family in terms of health care? What difference does it make? It is the patient who has the disease process! Why involve the family? Let us pause a moment to consider the nature of the health problems we are dealing with.

Victory Fuchs (1974), health economist, examined our national health care system and notes that medical advances beginning in the 1930s and extending through the 1950s have brought about significant improvements in health, especially through the control of infectious disease. For more than a decade, however, the impact of new medical discoveries on overall mortality has been slight. The chief killers today are heart disease, cancer, and especially for the young 15-24 years, automobile accidents, suicide and homicide. The behavioral component in all these causes of death is very large, and until now, medical care has not been very successful in altering behavior. Fuchs concludes:

> The greatest current potential for improving the health of the American people is to be found in what they do and don't do for themselves. Individual decisions about diet, exercise, and smoking are of critical importance.

This conference is principally relating to chronic and life-threatening pediatric illness. The treatment for many of these illnesses will take place over the entire life of the child and adolescent and, sometimes, on into adulthood. Recent medical advances have extended the life of many patients with serious illnesses such as childhood cancers and juvenile diabetes. How well that child and adolescent manages his or her chronic disease, experiences, and complies with the prescribed medical regimen depends a good deal on the patient's significant interpersonal relationships both within the natural family and with the professional health care family (Becker, 1975; Schultz, 1980).

PATIENT COMPLIANCE

Reviewing the literature about compliance with therapeutic regimens in pediatrics, Becker (1975) and Schultz (1980) found that poor family functioning seems to be rather consistently related to noncompliance. Pediatric clinic appointment breakers tended to come from disorganized families. Pediatric renal patients who are noncompliant tended to come from families with poor communications and dys-equilibrium. In relation to a rheumatic fever prevention program, it was found that poor participation seems to be related to family situations reflecting stresses such as marital separation, divorce, and conflicts that may have involved the police, psychiatric hospitalization, or a recent change of residence

(Schultz, 1980). The data suggest that pediatric patients from highly stressed or poorly functioning families may be at risk for problems in complying with therapeutic regimens. Simply having a diagnosis and knowing about the disease does not insure compliance.

In dealing with pediatric chronic disease and life-threatening illness, the family of the patient needs to be involved immediately in a truly integrated way with the professional health care givers who need to consider some of the following key issues: In what ways does the family of the ill child support and/or disrupt the treatment? What can be reasonably expected of the family in caring for the ill child? What is the effect on the well siblings? What are the emotional and financial sacrifices to be made by the family? Timing is very crucial in intervening with a family who is in crisis. Families sometimes may make decisions that may compound the severity of their situation. Appropriate and timely intervention may benefit the family (Kaplan, 1979).

HOME CARE

The importance of the family as a natural support system is seen, particularly, in reference to the economics of health care. Attention is increasingly being directed to an established, but still underused alternative--the home, an institution in its own right. A recent review of the findings of studies representative of the home health cost effectiveness found "home health care is indeed less expensive than extended hospitalization" (Hammond, 1979). Home care for some treatment regimens is also proving to be medically and emotionally advantageous to patients and their families. Major savings are also being cited in the national trend toward performing many surgical and medical procedures on an outpatient basis that once required hospitalization (Sullivan, 1980). For example, individuals with renal disease who undergo center-dialysis are often evaluated for home dialysis because the former is over twice the cost (Burton, 1977). Studies have shown that in home dialysis there is superior patient survival and improved rehabilitation (Whaler and Freeman, 1978; Burton, 1977). Martinson (1978) showed that not only is it feasible for families to care for dying children at home, but it is also much easier on the families' psychological adjustment and far less costly than hospital care. The children appeared to be relieved to be at home rather than in the hospital. They had their parents at hand, were surrounded by familiar furnishings, ate food that they were used to, and had the company of their siblings and pets. Finally, Martinson found "parents who take part in home care may return to normal sooner after the child's death...while they still grieved their child's death, they were able to resume their normal work duties sooner than the parents of patients who died in the hospital" (Martinson, 1978).

Clearly, there appear to be advantages in home care for some medical conditions. However, there are many seriously ill children and adults where the family would be too disrupted psychologically, physically, and financially to undertake the care of the ill member (Litman, 1979). With greater interest in home care, research needs to be carried out to evaluate its appropriateness and feasibility for a variety of medical problems.

CONCLUSION

In summary, I have attempted to highlight the timeliness of this symposium within a clinical, a societal, a humanitarian, and an economic context. The ideas, concepts, and clinical illustrations presented will be an opportunity to weigh and consider the value and contribution of the natural and the professional health care family in understanding and treating chronic and life-threatening pediatric medical illness.

The interactional and systems viewpoint attempts to put problems on a human scale and in terms of joint responsibility. Therefore, as we discern significant relationships between interaction and physical illness, we are up against the issue of responsibility for these problems. As Weakland (1977) notes and cautions, "Any positive findings about interaction and disease might well, at least initially be seen more as accusations that people are making their loved ones sick; than as a realistic and helpful recognition of how, even without benefit of ceremony, we are in life together, for better or worse, in sickness and in health, until death do us part--and sometimes even beyond. "

REFERENCES

American Medical Association. National Commission on the Cost of Medical Care 1976-77. Munroe, Wisconsin, 1978.
Becker, M. H. and Green, W. W. A Family Approach to Compliance with Medical Treatment. International Journal of Health Education, 18, 2-11, 1975.
Bell, J. E. The Family in the Hospital: Lessons from Developing Countries. Chevy Chase, Maryland. National Institute of Mental Health, 1969.
Bell, J. E. Family Therapy. New York: Jason Aronsen, 1975.
Bloch, D. A. The Family of the Psychiatric Patient. In S. Arieti (Ed.) American Handbook of Psychiatry, New York: Basic Books, 1974.
Burton, B. T. The Federal Government and Home Hemodialysis. Journal of Dialysis, 5, 457-463, 1977.
Cooper, D. The Death of the Family, New York: Pantheon, 1971.
Fuchs, V. Who Shall Live? Health, Economics and Social Choice, New York: Basic Books, 1974.

Gartner, A. and Riessman, F. Self-Help in the Human Services.
    San Francisco: Jossey-Bass, 1977.
Grolnick, L. A Family Perspective of Psychosomatic Factors in Ill-
    ness: A Review of the Literature. Family Process, 11, 457-486,
    1972.
Hammond, J. Home Health Care Cost Effectiveness: An Overview of
    the Literature. Public Health Reports, 94, 305-311, 1979.
Kaplan, D. M. and Grandstaff, N. A Problem Solving Approach to
    Terminal Illness for the Family and Physician. In C. Garfield
    (Ed.) Stress and Survival. St. Louis: C. V. Mosby & Company,
    1979.
Knowles, J. H. Doing Better and Feeling Worse: Health in the United
    States. In E. G. Jaco (Ed.) Patients Physicians and Illness,
    New York: The Free Press, 1979.
Litman, T. J. The Family in Health and Health Care: A Social-
    Behavioral Overview. In E. G. Jaco (Ed.) Patients, Physicians
    and Illness. New York: The Free Press, 1979.
Martinson, I. M., Armstrong, G. D. Home Care for Children Dying
    of Cancer. Pediatrics, 62, 106-113, 1978.
Mauksch, H. O. A Social Science Basis for Conceptualizing Famil-
    Health. Social Science and Medicine, 8, 521-528, 1974.
McWhinney, I. S. Family Medicine in Perspective. The New England
    Journal of Medicine, 293, 176-180, 1975.
Meissner, W. W. Family Dynamics and Psychosomatic Processes.
    Family Process, 5, 142-161, 1966.
Powles, J. On the Limitations of Modern Medicine. In D. S. Sobel
    (Ed.) Ways of Health. New York: Harcourt, Brace, Jovanovich,
    1979.
Ruzek, S. B. The Women's Health Movement. New York: Praeger, 1978.
Schultz, S. K. Compliance with Therapeutic Regimens in Pediatrics:
    A Review of Implications for Social Work Practice. Social
    Work in Health Care, 5, 267-278, 1980.
Shapiro, J. Changing Dysfunctional Relationships Between Family and
    Hospital. Journal of Operational Psychiatry, 11, 18-26, 1980.
Sobel, D. S. Ways of Health. New York: Harcourt, Brace Jovanovich,
    1979.
Sullivan, R. Outpatient Surgery. The New York Times, November 22,
    1980.
Weakland, J. H. "Family Somatics" A Neglected Edge. Family Process,
    16, 263-272, 1977.
Whalen, J. E. and Freeman, R. M. Home Hemodialysis Review in Iowa
    1970-1977. Archives of Internal Medicine, 138, 178-190, 1978.

FAMILY TREATMENT OF CHRONIC ILLNESS IN A CHILD: MUTUAL DEVELOPMENTAL
PROBLEMS

Irving N. Berlin, M.D.

University of New Mexico School of Medicine

Albuquerque, New Mexico

INTRODUCTION

Development has only recently been thought of as a continuum,
both in children and adults, throughout the entire life cycle
(Erikson, 1963). There have been a number of papers which recognize that parenthood is an important developmental phase, not
previously discussed until Theresa Benedek (1959) and others pointed
out that adult development is especially affected by marriage and
parenthood, and that failures in development are important issues to
be examined in the treatment of adults. It has been our experience,
in working with disorganized families, that one of the major obstacles in helping a family towards more integrative behavior is the
failure in development in both parents. This failure is threatened
as each of their children begins to develop and approach a more
successful resolution of developmental tasks than one or the other
or both of the parents have yet experienced. Often such developmental attainments in the children are, in part, due to the greater
maturity of one parent or a special interest in a child by a teacher
or another adult in the child's life (Berlin, 1979; Anthony, 1973;
Anthony and Benedek, 1970).

In therapeutic work with children, adolescents and parents, the
child's progress may be impeded if one cannot simultaneously help
the parents towards more effective functioning. Viewed from a
developmental standpoint, when severe disorders of childhood and
adolescence occur, similar to the patients described in the case
reports that follow, there has to be interrelated developmental
movement in similar areas by both child and parents.

Normative Developmental Crises in the Child

The achievement of normal developmental stages in a child's life may depend upon whether the parents have had major problems and conflicts in passing through those stages. (Problems of any severity in the stage of bonding and attachment have such pervasive effects and are so fundamental to development that they are not discussed in this context.) The beginning individuation and separation which occurs between two and four years of age, with autonomous strivings and the earlier development of object constancy occurs as the child learns to master both the use of his limbs and the use of speech. The separation and individuation process may pose problems for parents who have nurtured the child. They are faced with the developmental momentum toward separation and leaving the parents, especially mother, which may interfere with their needs for a dependent, loving and nurturing child. The nursery school or day care situation often highlights these problems. The child's eagerness to begin to learn and to utilize its curiosity and investigativeness for acquiring new knowledge is also a focus in separation from the mother in the primary grades. During this phase of normal development, the parents are confronted with the fact that peers and other adults become important parts of the child's world, as the child continues to learn and become an effective individual. Those parents who have not themselves developed through these stages of interest in learning and developing exciting peer and other adult relationships may need to block such separation and individuation efforts (Anthony, 1973).

Parental Failures in Development--Effect on Child

Throughout the growth of the child, as developmental stages are reached and the child seeks to master them, the parents' failure in mastery of a particular developmental stage may prevent that child from effectively mastering the same stage. If the child is fortunate enough to have extra-familial experiences which allow this development, the child's beginning to master a particular stage often presents serious conflicts for the parents. It thus seems as if most children are destined to repeat the developmental failures of their parents. From time to time, we see developmental crises which result from the parents' inability to deal with a developmental need or drive of the child. We also see a similar phenomenon in treatment, where working through developmental arrests or delays by the child depends on the parents being helped to resolve developmental problems from similar phases.

The clearest failures in parental development which adversely affect the child occur in child abuse. Parents who have not been nurtured in infancy, who have been neglected or abused during the period of striving for autonomy and the development of curiosity

and investigativeness, and have never been responded to as a child
who needs to play, remain fixed in development with the constant
need for nurturance for themselves. When they are faced by their
own child who begins to walk, talk and to investigate the world,
such parents may see such investigation and striving for autonomy
as deliberate and malicious, deserting the parent and ignoring the
parents' needs. They attribute to the two-year-old child the adult
capacity for understanding directions and commands. They have no
understanding of a child's developmental need to play, to investigate, or to be nurtured. Child abuse, therefore, often comes about
as the child's developmental needs and drives impinge upon the
parents' needs. The parents become harsh, intimidating, and finally
assaultive if the child is not responsive to them as a little adult.
Having never resolved these developmental issues themselves, they
have no way of understanding the child's developmental needs and
fostering them. Thus, the violence in their own lives at a similar
age is passed on to their children as they begin to develop (Steele,
1970).

Parental Learning and Child Learning

Another area of developmental failure of parents which is
frequently manifested, occurs in the areas of learning. This is
most readily seen in the school setting. Parents who have not had
very much encouragement to learn and attend school and have not had
the opportunity to develop their own curiosity and to be stimulated
by learning, do not have much concern with their child's learning.
There is a good deal of data both from the Headstart studies, the
work of Weikert (1968) and other educators and from the Plowden
Report (1966) in England which indicates that, regardless of socio-
economic class, the single most important factor in the success of
a child in school is the parents' attitudes towards the child's
learning.

It is also clear that some parents, whose children have been
influenced by teachers who have become important to their development, may resent their children's learning because they themselves
have not learned. In several experimental projects, efforts have
been made to help the parents to learn along with the children so
that the ideas acquired by the children are not totally foreign to
the parents. The parents, therefore, become concerned with the
child's learning and pleased with the child's accomplishments
(Berlin and Berlin, 1975).

Developmental Issues and Specific Developmental Lines

One developmental crises is related to cognitive development
and to the fact that, in early adolescence, there is a shift from
concrete operations to formal operations in those youngsters where

there has been preparation for formal operational thought. This
new capacity to generate hypotheses, to think about problem solving
in new and creative ways, to become excited by the reasoning in
science and mathematics, history or philosophy, and also learn to
deal with the world around oneself in new and innovative ways, may
also disturb parents who still function at concrete operational
levels. Many adolescents never reach formal operational thinking
due to little encouragement or lack of adult models.

Developmental Issues of Independence and Intimacy

     During the period of adolescence, with the surge of sexual
feelings, there are needs for independence and for development of
intimate relations with individuals of the same and opposite sex.
Parents who have not been able to achieve both independence and
intimacy are still bound to their own parents. They are not able
to free their children to explore and become independent. These
parents have never been able to experience actual intimacy. They
look for nurturance throughout their lives from their own spouses,
but are never able to actually achieve it, hence find themselves in
constant conflict with the child who is making these developmental
strides. The violent feelings of adults towards the adolescent may
represent anger that they will be replcaced by someone who is, in
many ways, going to experience life and relationships in ways that
the parents have hoped to experience but have not been able to.
Tuus, the adolescent's strivings towards more successful experiences
in intimacy, sexuality, a new work role and financial success may
all cause parental disturbances, anger, and family conflict because
the parents have not worked through these adolescent developmental
stages successfully (Anthony, 1969).

Psychotic and Severe Psychosomatic Disorders and Developmental Issues for Parents

     In each of these disorders, most clearly noted in a number of
psychosomatic disorders, as the child is helped to overcome a
depression or reduce the intensity of a psychosomatic disorder and
to continue to progress in areas where development had previously
been arrested, simultaneous treatment of parents is necessary to
prevent parental interferences with their child's development in
their desperate effort to retain the status quo. Parents may be
threatened by their child's developmental gains as reminders of their
own failures in development as previously noted (Minuchin, 1970;
Gardner, 1969; Mattson and Agle, 1972).

Case Vignette: A Child with Asthma

     Perry, at age 9, had had severe asthma for three years. His
parents and two older siblings, Anne, age 14, and Paul, age 16,

lived in constant terror of his severe attacks, which always occurred
in the middle of the night and precipitated a family emergency,
such as hustling Perry to the County Hospital Emergency for Adrenalin
injections and oxygen.

Somehow, there was never a warning of these attacks. Also,
despite Perry's severe allergic reactions to many airborne plant
and flower pollens, and to dog and cat danders, the family always
seemed to have several stray cats around which had been brought home
by Perry or his brother. This occurred despite the pediatric
allergist's strict injunctions against such animals in the house.
Though the house was kept scrupulously clean, and parents or
siblings took Perry regularly for his desensitization injections,
his midnight asthmatic attacks and occasional status asthmaticus
continued to increase in frequency.

Perry was referred to the child psychiatric clinic by the school
teacher and counselor, with the enthusiastic endorsement of the
pediatrician, because of increased wheezing in the classroom and
attacks of asthma which kept him out of school as he approached any
test. Though he was a good reader, he began to wheeze during any
reading test, especially when being tested for comprehension. He
had his worst attacks prior to arithmetic tests. Thus, he was
failing in most subjects despite good intelligence and clear evidence
of a capacity to learn.

His parents, Joe and Sally, both in their early forties, were
raised in the rural Midwest by very strict authoritarian and religious parents, who were quite punitive. Both came from large •
families, each with a history of severe mental illness in their
extended families. When they married and moved to the west coast,
they were determined to be "kindly" parents. For five years they
avoided having children and enjoyed their life together. With
their first child, Paul, a very active baby, they found themselves
quite angry at the child and estranged from each other, since their
whole life was disrupted. As this information emerged during
couples therapy, it became clear that although they were not harsh
or punitive parents, they found it difficult to be giving and loving
in face of their children's needs and demands. They had their
second child as "company for the first." Anne was a placid girl,
easier for mother to care for and for father to relate to. Since
the parents had played little as children, they did not play with
their own children. Both parents bemoaned the fact that their life
was never as intimate and pleasurable after their children's births.

Perry's birth was an accident; they had decided not to have
any more children. Perry was a colicky, difficult baby who slept
little, ate poorly and gained little weight. Mother recalls her
constant anger at him because he could never be quieted, and

disturbed everyone's sleep. Both siblings were expected to take
care of him when home from school.

Perry's asthma coincided with his entering the first grade.
In kindergarten, he had a very warm, caring teacher, and he seemed
to blossom. He had the usual frequent colds and constant runny
nose, but began to make friends and was less complaining and ate
better at home. In the first grade, without any favorite status,
he appeared less happy and had his first severe asthma attack with
a severe cold.

Only after six months of family and couples therapy did
mother and father begin to recall his asthma-like attacks in the
first and second years of life, when each cold led to severe difficulties in breathing, requiring steam tents and medication. Their
physician said he would grow out of it.

In our first interviews with the parents, it was clear that
Perry was not the only problem at home. Paul was experiencing
learning and behavior problems in school, mostly "a short fuse,"
with a violent temper. Anne was a good student but had a long
period of refusing to attend school in the first three grades.
Mother could not force herself to take her and leave her in school,
until threatened with a court hearing. Mother felt Anne was sickly
and needed to be with her at home. Mother also used her to keep
Perry company. Father, a skilled tool and die maker, became very
much involved in his fraternal order and was rarely at home, which
caused constant bickering between the parents.

In the playroom, Perry first was very withdrawn and ignored
all the toys. When I finally encouraged him to play dominoes with
me and he won, he looked frightened. When I laughingly complimented
him on his good playing, he relaxed slightly. As I modeled playful
anger at him when he blocked me or was winning, or gloated openly
when I was ahead, he would look at me half-scared. In a few weeks
he imitated my mock anger and would whisper "stinker" when I was
winning. After an unusual run of good luck on my part and my goading
him that he'd never win a game, he screamed out "you S.O.B." and
looked very frightened. At my easy acceptance of his feelings and
after I placed the inflated Bobo punching bag next to us so we could
each slug him when we felt angry, he gradually began to express
anger both in physical action and in words. It was more difficult
for him to gloat over me when he was winning, but gradually he
began to do this. After five months of weekly sessions, his
wheezing was infrequent, and when it did occur, it disappeared as
he ventilated either anger at my winning or pleasure at my troubles.
He would react to my dramatic modeling of both anger or glee with
an almost patronizing warm smile, recognizing the encouraging,
supportive intent of my dramatic behavior to help promote his more

open expression of feelings.

In their couples therapy, the parents found it very difficult to discuss their current problems. When I began to ask them to describe in detail the parallels between how they understood and interacted with their children as compared to their parents' behavior towards them, both of the parents felt they were more understanding and helpful to their children than their parents had been toward them. The details of their own childhood experiences led to a discussion of their children's views of them. In our early family sessions, only their daughter, Anne, viewed either parent as supportive, encouraging, or warm. All the children seemed to feel that father had been isolating himself from the family, and that mother always seemed too busy with housework to listen to the children's problems. Both parents protested that while those feelings might be how they were viewed, their children were still treated better than they had been. I acknowledged this as true, and wondered if they did not want their children to view them as having been supportive. I knew it was hard to practice what they had not experienced, but felt they had the desire and wanted to be more effective as parents. After the parents explored how they saw their partner in his or her role with the children and confirmed the views of their children, I suggested we try to find tasks that each could carry out with their two boys to enhance their ability to function both at home and in school. I suggested a family meeting to discuss these tasks. Both parents reluctantly agreed to another family meeting, feeling coerced by Perry's most recent asthmatic attack, yet hoping to find some relief from the anxiety brought on by these attacks. In the family meeting, Paul said he had always admired his dad's skill with tools, but father always ignored his offer to help with the auto repairs. While father admitted that he hated onlookers when he worked, he would be willing to try to teach Paul how to do engine tune-ups. We asked Paul to try to restrain himself and not walk out if he could not do a task the first time. Father smiled and said he would try not to be too impatient. Mother, who had been an "A" student through high school because of encouraging teachers, volunteered to work with Perry to complete some math assignments. Perry looked frightened and said it made him scared to think of mother looking over his shoulder, and he began to wheeze. However, he agreed to try if mother would not demand he be perfect. Mother sighed with tension and said she would try. Anne said she knew mother could be helpful, and she would try to help Perry with his social studies.

We were clearly asking each parent to try to be more nurturing with their children and asking the young people to try to accept such efforts without too much anger or resistance.

We had weekly family meetings over the next ten weeks to focus

on problems in carrying out these tasks. Father and Paul each had
several blow-ups with the other. When we examined these in detail,
we could pinpoint father's expectations that Paul know some aspects
of engine mechanics, and Paul's difficulty in listening as father
tried to explain something. Over a period of weeks, Paul began to
say he did not understand something, and father would go over it
again. Father began to explain in greater detail the basic function
of various engine parts. When Paul succeeded in doing a complete
tune-up, he and father celebrated by going out for a pizza together.

When father had a big job at the Lodge and needed to get out
some mimeographed fliers, he asked Paul to help. Paul did so
with some reluctance. Though it was a boring job for Paul to do the
collating, he quickly learned how to run the machine, which pleased
father. Father, who was one of the Lodge's best bowlers, was helped
in a family session to agree to try to teach Paul to bowl, though
Paul initially protested that he was not interested. To father's
amazement, Paul was very athletic, had a good eye, and learned
quickly. Father bragged that those skills came from his side of the
family. After a poor frame, when Paul wanted to slam the ball down
on the alley, father angrily restrained him and then showed him
where his footwork was sloppy.

When mother began to protest that the car repairs and bowling
kept Paul and father away from home more than ever, they agreed
during a family meeting to make bowling a family affair, with
dinner out, which placated mother a bit. Stormy as the interactions
between father and Paul were, mother and Perry had many very anxious
interactions, with several frightening asthmatic attacks interrupting
their studying together. In the family meetings, Anne began to
describe some moments when she happened to be close by and witnessed
mother trying to help Perry with a math assignment. As mother im-
patiently tried to help Perry understand a concept, he began to make
errors and was wheezing slightly. Rather than stopping at that
point and giving Perry his Tedral and Adrenalin mist, they continued
the lesson until Perry had a full-blown attack. With Anne's help,
mother would listen to the wheezing, stop, and minister to Perry.
After things calmed down, they would work for a short time again.
Perry seemed much more relaxed after mother took care of him and
seemed more attentive to her instructions. Finally, mother could
ask Perry to tell her when he felt pressured, and she would try to
help him in another way. Mother began to notice Perry's anxious
frown when he felt pressured, and would stop their lesson. Perry
began to let mother know when he felt pushed. It was clear in our
sessions that Perry very much looked forward to working with his
mother. He had little trouble with Anne's helping him, both because
he was better at social studies and because Anne, very intuitively,
made their work into a learning game, which Perry enjoyed.

As the family members began to function more cohesively, the

asthma disrupted their lives to a lesser degree; there were fewer
calls from school about Paul's behavior problems, and Anne's problems
came into focus, as did the parents' interpersonal problems.

Anne, a blossoming adolescent girl, began to find herself
attractive to many boys and attracted to several of them. When
she contemplated dating one of them, she began to have severe stomach
aches, which reminded her of her sick stomach when she was unable
to leave mother and attend the first grade. In a series of sessions
with Anne and her parents, the issues of sexuality and sex education
were discussed. Mother and father helped her to understand that
it was alright to begin to step out into the world on her own. They
talked about the differences between sexual desire and love and
intimacy, how she would learn that, and what expectations they had
of Anne and her future as a young person who needed to become
independent, to leave home, find a work role, a partner in living,
etc.

This exploration opened up many of the parents' current
difficulties with each other. In couple sessions they explored
their pleasures in intimacy, sex and togetherness during the first
years of their marriage. Their life together had never been the
same since Paul's birth. As they were helped to talk out what was
best for Anne, mother (who had never read a book on sex education)
agreed that she and father should read The Joys of Sex by Comfort,
so they could both answer Anne's questions. They also requested
a book for Anne and previewed it so mother and Anne could talk
together. Father recognized that he had never talked to Paul
directly about sex, but had been discussing girl friends with him
when they were alone. He felt Paul and he should also read the
same book so they could talk together.

Reading The Joys of Sex led the parents to go off to a friend's
mountain cabin for a weekend to try to alter their infrequent and
perfunctory sexual relations. They came back looking younger and
very shy. Mother wasn't sure she could really talk about sex with
Anne, but said she would try. They gave both their adolescents
permission to attend the school classes on physical and psychological aspects of parenthood, which also discussed reproduction and
sexual concerns of young people.

Thus, through the seven months of family and couples therapy,
and while dealing with Anne's adolescent developmental needs, both
parents dealt with their own adolescent issues. They were able to
decide that they could use some of their savings to help either
Paul or Anne or both to obtain the college education they never had,
which they had never thought about before. This family made many
strides, and each child began to develop more normally. Perry's
asthma ceased and Paul's acting up slowly dissipated. Anne was

allowed to individuate, as was Paul, and both parents grew as parents, as individuals and as more loving adults in their marriage.

Case Vignette: A Case of Colitis

Steve was first seen in the hospital on the surgical ward at age 15. He was being considered for a colostomy. The nurses were so angry at his vicious verbal attacks on them that they feared their avoidance of him and frequent errors in giving medication would result in Steve's death. They prevailed upon the surgeons for a psychiatric consultation.

Steve was hostile to the consultant, calling him obscene names, saying no "shrink" could help him. These comments were understood in terms of his own rage, his feelings of helplessness, hopelessness, and of being unloved. His parents rarely visited because he screamed and cursed at them. When the child psychiatrist suggested a family conference, Steve sneered, "no one would come." The frightened parents did come. It was clear from this meeting that Steve's early life had been one of great maternal neglect. His step-mother came into the family one year after Steve's mother died of uterine cancer following two years of illness. Steve was five years old at the time. Father's depression precluded much nurturance of Steve during that crucial three year period. After a series of babysitters, by the time his father remarried, Steve believed no one cared about him. His hostility and demandingness quickly alienated him from his step-mother and father, and from anyone else who interacted with him. At age eight, his illness and symptoms were first diagnosed as colitis, and were always treated medically. His parents always felt helpless in dealing with Steve's illness and with his hostile, difficult behavior.

The parents were asked to visit Steve three times a week for fifteen minutes each time. If need be, they could sit and read in order to be able to withstand Steve's tirades. This first request to the parents was designed to help them feel more parental and to give Steve a sense that they cared about him. Nurses were also helped to recognize Steve's anger as a challenge to determine if someone could care for such a horrible person (Plank, 1971).

After four weeks of interminable testing, Steve was convinced his efforts could not drive his parents, the nurses, or his therapist away. Steve was then asked if he "was man enough" to try to take enough fluids by mouth to make I.V.'s unnecessary. It seemed likely it would be hard to do this. He responded sarcastically that if his parents could stand him, he would try to drink more fluids. Though not totally successful, it was an important step for Steve to try and help himself. He was, however, still hostile, rejecting the people who tried to spend time with him. He derided my approving comments that he had tried to take fluids orally. Since most of his abuse was aimed at his step-mother, we felt it would be she who might be most helpful to him and suggested a mutual task. Mother was a school teacher and Steve was a failure in school. We asked mother to pick some science fiction stories to read to Steve, and we asked Steve to see if he would concentrate enough on the story to be able to repeat the main points. We realized both his physical pain and his anger at his step-mother would make it difficult. She was in tears after her first attempt. He had called her foul names and made obscene comments about every character in the story. Her only relief occurred when the nurse came in to give him broth and jello, which he consumed with relish. When we commented on this successful outcome of her task, she laughed and for the first time was able to understand Steve's great hunger for concern and attention, and his anger at not being loved and nurtured by anyone. During the next week, the derision continued. However, the day before the family meeting, Steve offhandedly and mockingly said to his step-mother that it was a child's task to retell the plot of the story read to him. He then did it.

With his therapist, Steve kept up a railing, hostile banter. He would, however, respond to the therapist's humorous and empathetic comments with some smiling and a "see you next time, Doc" at the end of each daily 30 minute session.

We turned to father next to try and help him reduce his helplessness with Steve. Steve tolerated his visits in a sullen silence. Father's regular tri-weekly visits resulted in a reduction of the verbal abuse. It was father to whom Steve used to turn as a child when his gut was in turmoil and he was beginning to have massive diarrhea. Father would then suggest they go to the hospital to stop the diarrhea and fluid loss. Steve, even at ages 8-10, would stubbornly refuse or have a raging temper tantrum. Father would helplessly give in until Steve was so dehydrated that it became an acute emergency and he was taken, protesting weakly, to the hospital. Father had never been able to be firm and authoritative. We asked father to spend his visits with Steve talking about his dilemmas when Steve was young, being frank about his need to be liked, about his fear of asserting himself and having Steve hate him for spending so little time with him, and about how depressed, shaky and indecisive his wife's illness and death had left him. Father had previously talked with the therapist about his acute depression and subsequent guilt when he ignored Steve's needs. Father had taken care of his own needs when he remarried, and was surprised at Steve's rejection of the step-mother. Father had ignored Steve's hostile attacks on him, his belligerent behavior in school, and their pediatrician's concern with Steve's beginning bowel problems, gut aches, and long periods of diarrhea. Only the first prolonged bout of illness and Steve's hospitalization made him guiltily aware of how little attention he had given Steve.

Father, after some rehearsal with the therapist, was able to describe to Steve his feelings during mother's last years of illness and death. At first, Steve would scream at father and interrupt him. Given encouragement to persist, father found that Steve's protests grew more feeble, and he could make his voice heard above Steve's derisive comments. By the middle of the second week of these efforts, Steve listened quietly but with evident discomfort. He was especially uneasy and upset when father wept while describing his feelings on mother's death and later his feelings of defeat and uncertainty about asserting himself with his son, feeling his son hated him. Steve's frequent interruptions to call the nurse to attend to him were difficult for father. However, this led to the first honest exchange of feelings about how father felt on being interrupted as he talked to his son. Steve's response was, "you scare me; I don't know how to deal with your feelings."

Progressively, the tasks suggested to Steve and his parents reflected the shifts in their adaptive capacities and mutual development. These new behaviors were decided on in the family sessions, both in terms of what Steve could agree he needed, and what each family member was ready for. Thus, step-mother was psychologically ready to begin a basic tutoring program with Steve. This was a sign of her greater maturity. While her original reason for marrying was to find a kindly figure from whom she could derive care and whose great needs permitted her to be nurturing without being overwhelmed, she did not plan to encounter a raging, unsatisfiable child, and was so overwhelmed that she finally withdrew. At this point, she and father were more open about their feelings, were mutually supportive and had learned they could withstand Steve's rages without having to run away or counterattack. Both had grown considerably in their couples therapy. Thus, mother was ready to work with Steve weeks before Steve could consider exposing his lack of basic academic skills. Both Steve and step-mother agreed on an interim period of reading of elementary U. S. history, especially the revolutionary and civil wars, which Steve was interested in but could not yet read easily. As Steve gained weight and his diarrhea subsided, Steve and father talked more freely about their memories around the time of mother's death. We agreed that they should make a visit from the hospital to mother's grave. They appeared more relaxed and closer to each other on return, and Steve, for the first time, evidenced interest in his father's sports car. He said he would love to learn to drive it.

We tried to help Steve and father to determine when Steve was well enough and father secure enough for Steve to get his learner's permit. A month later they began to use passes from the hospital for father to teach Steve to drive the family car, much to Steve's disappointment. After a prolonged and acrimonious debate about the fact that he did not need to learn to drive a regular car first and that he was being treated as a baby, he reacted to father's firmness about the sequence of learning to drive with good grace. It was clear father had learned to be more parental, to use his best judgment no matter how much hostile opposition he got from Steve.

By the time Steve was released from the hospital to outpatient care in Surgery and Child-Adolescent Psychiatry, there was no need for a colostomy. Steve had accepted the tutoring and step-mother could end Steve's stormy tirades when he did poorly by being very clear and firm and ending the lesson, returning to it the next day. Steve discovered, to his dismay, that his coordination was not very good. He gradually learned to drive the family car, and worked with the physical therapist to enhance his strength and sensorimotor integration.

Thus, over a period of almost five months, Steve improved from an emaciated, hostile, bitter candidate for colostomy to a 16 year old ready to deal both with his old problems, the grief about the loss of his mother, and his overwhelming need to be nurtured and accepted uncritically, no matter how he behaved. As both father and stepmother could be nondefensively firm in the face of Steve's irrational demands and clarify what they believed was reasonable, Steve's demands diminished. He then gradually began to deal with his problems of adolescence with parents, peers and educators. He was essentially asymptomatic for colitis. Steve's retarded psycho-social, cognitive and social development were gradually worked on in both individual and family therapy. The parents developed as they continued their therapeutic work. They acknowledged that they found themselves better able to be honest with each other. Their relationship flourished.

SUMMARY AND CONCLUSIONS

Only in the past decade has human psychological development been viewed as a continuous process from birth through old age. Benedek (1959) and others have emphasized the developmental impact of parenthood. Erikson (1963) has defined specific developmental tasks for each stage.

Work with a variety of families, most obvious in disorganized or dysfunctional families, reveals that every developmental stage lived through by a child in a family may result in parental anxiety, tension, anger and retaliatory behavior if one or both of them has had major delays or interferences in completing the developmental tasks of that stage. Much child abuse can be related to the needs of the small child, revealing failures in the parents' development in being nurtured, in developing good object relations and in individuating from their parents. Oedipal problems are manifested both during that period but especially during adolescence. Pubertal changes, normal sexual interest in young people of the opposite sex, and development of close peer relations all evoke retaliatory anger and anxiety in parents who have failed to work through earlier stages in their own development, with resulting mutual sexual dissatisfactions. Much strife occurs due to the independent strivings of the young person. The achievement of closeness and intimacy in the adolescent's relations with others may be interfered with by the anxieties, possessiveness and jealousies of parents who yearn for but have never themselves achieved these developmental goals.

In treatment of severely disturbed adolescents, with depression, psychosis or severe psychophysiologic disturbance, the milieu program, group, individual and family therapy are aimed at helping the adolescent make up for some of the past developmental failures and begin to address the current adolescent tasks.

The work with the family engages all members in first recognizing the developmental goals of adolescence. Then a task-oriented plan is developed to help the parents promote various stages of adolescent development. The adolescent is helped to collaborate in these efforts. In this process, parents also begin to overcome some of their developmental delays as they are helped to encourage their adolescent's development by carrying out specific parental tasks.

In the first case illustration, both parents were helped to work through oedipal problems as their adolescent son and daughter began to deal with these issues. Earlier problems of separation and individuation were also worked on as the child in the playroom worked through his anger at the lack of parental nurturance and anxiety about becoming independent from mother. As both parents slowly succeeded in their assigned parental tasks with both sons, they found it easier to be more openly supportive and nurturant to their children and still allow them distance and individuality. Issues of sexuality, intimacy, closeness and independence came into focus as the parents were helped to deal with their daughter's adolescent crushes. In that process, they recaptured some of their early intimacy and mutual sexual pleasure. They were able to help Anne and then Paul to separate more easily from them, since the parents experienced more tenderness and closeness with each other.

The second case deals with severe ulcerative colitis in an adolescent, resulting at least in part from the death of the mother when the patient was about four years old. It is clear that mother's earlier illness precluded much nurturance. Father abandoned his parental role both because of his own depression at his wife's death and his guilt at not being able to respond to his son's needs for nurturance. His son's hostility prevented father from requiring that he get treatment early, with resulting serious illnesses and repeated hospitalizations.

In the face of a possible colostomy, a total treatment program, including step-mother and father in family therapy and individual psychotherapy for the adolescent was begun. This malignantly hostile adolescent was gradually able to experience and understand the caring attitude of his parents, therapists, and nurses as they stayed with him through his bitter tirades. Each parent was given tasks to work on with their son to establish trust and to enhance his competence as an adolescent. Finally, father's ability to honestly describe his confusion and failure to help his son when he was young, despite his son's angry efforts not to hear, proved to be a major breakthrough.

In individual psychotherapy, a number of issues relating to fear of abandonment, of being able to accept caring from others, as well as working through oedipal feelings towards his step-mother occurred. This permitted some of the early adolescent tasks to be worked on, as he began to feel competent and independent, without anxiety about being abandoned. As father was more clearly and unambivalently paternal, the irrational demands of his son decreased. Both parents learned to be more straightforward with each other as they learned how important honesty was to their son. Thus, their relationship improved in every sphere, including the sexual one.

Many parents are unable to continue their development as adults because of their earlier developmental delays due to severe deprivation in infancy and early childhood. Sometimes, overwhelming life events interfere with parents' continued development during critical phases of a child's life, which stunts both the child's and parents' development.

In a number of cases we have been able to help children, adolescents, and their parents utilize the crises which brought them to treatment to gradually overcome some previous developmental problems. When such progress occurs, the child is freed to make up for previous developmental delays and to resume and work through the current issues in development. Parents may make up some of their developmental deficits with mutual conflict reduction and improvement in living of all family members.

REFERENCES

Anthony, E. J. The Reaction of Adults to Adolescents and their Behavior. In: G. Caplan and S. Lebovici (Eds.), Adolescence. New York:Basic Books, 1969.
Anthony, E. J. and Benedek, T. Parenthood: Its Psychology and Psychopathology. Boston: Little Brown and Co., pp. 449-477, 1970.

Anthony, E. J. A Working Model for Family Studies: A Developmental-
    Transactional Model. In: E. J. Anthony and C. Koupernik (Eds.),
    The Child in His Family: The Impact of Disease and Death.
    New York: John Wiley and Sons, pp. 3-20, 1973.
Benedek, T. Parenthood as a Developmental Phase: A Contribution
    to the Libido Therapy. Journal of the American Psychoanalytic
    Association, 7, 389-417, 1959.
Berlin, I. N. and Berlin, R. Parents on the Developmental Advocates
    of Children. In: I. N. Berlin (Ed.), Advocacy for Child Mental
    Health, New York: Brunner-Mazel, pp. 37-45, 1975.
Berlin, I. N. A Developmental Approach to Work with Disorganized
    Families. Journal of the American Academy of Child Psychiatry,
    18, (2), pp. 354-365, 1979.
Erikson, E. H. Eight Ages of Man. In: E. H. Erikson, (Ed.),
    Childhood and Society, New York: W. W. Norton and Company,
    pp. 247-274, 1963.
Gardner, R. The Guilt Reaction of Parents of Children with Severe
    Physical Disease. American Journal of Psychiatry, 126:5, 1969.
Mattson, A. and Agle, D. P. Group Therapy with Parents of Hemo-
    pheliacs: Therapeutic Process and Observations of Parental
    Adaptations to Chronic Illness in Children. Journal of
    American Academy of Child Psychiatry, 11:558-571, 1972.
Minuchin, S. The Use of an Ecological Framework in Treatment of
    a Child. In: E. J. Anthony and C. Koupernik (Eds.), The Child
    in His Family, New York: Wiley Interscience, pp. 41-58, 1970.
Plank, Emma N. Working with Children in Hospitals. Chicago: Year
    Book Medical Publishers, 1971.
Plowden Report: Central Advisory Council for Education (England):
    Children and Their Primary Schools, Vol. 1. London: Her
    Majesty's Stationery Office, 1966.
Steele, B. F. Parental Abuse of Infants and Small Children.
    In: E. J. Anthony and T. Benedek (Eds.), Parenthood: Its
    Psychology and Psychopathology, Boston: Little Brown, pp. 449-
    477, 1970.
Weikert, D. and Lambie, D. Preschool Intervention Through a Home
    Teaching Program. In: J. Hellmuth (Ed.), Disadvantaged Child,
    Vol. 2, New York: Brunner-Mazel, pp. 435-500, 1968.

FAMILY TREATMENT IS HERE TO STAY: DISCUSSION OF DR. BERLIN'S PAPER

Åke Mattsson, M. D.

New York University Medical Center

New York, New York

Dr. Berlin emphasizes how mutual developmental problems in a family may impair a child's coping with chronic illness. Without stressing it, he is applying an open systems model to family inter-action. He also is alluding to the normative critical stages of adult and family development.

Dr. Berlin stresses how often therapeutic work with children cannot succeed unless the family can be helped to function more effectively. Indeed, it is true that many children are destined to repeat problems during specific developmental stages much like their parents. This might be particularly striking in those children who cannot negotiate the individuation-separation phase because of their parents' difficulties to let go of their toddlers. We may see a prolongation of close inter-dependence between mother, father, and child, a fact that frequently seems related to later development of borderline personality organization.

With regard to the adolescent's shift from concrete to formal operations, we are struck by its significance for chronically ill and handicapped adolescents. They learn how to conceptualize their illness and life situation in a broader and deeper way, i.e. com-paring themselves to other ill youngsters, speculating about their future, using deductive-hypothetical reasoning to reason from the past to future possibilities. This helps them cope with their physical and psychological problems in a new way. If the parents of these adolescents are unable to operate cognitively on an abstract level, and only think "concretely", this may cause family conflicts. Simply speaking, the adolescent may be ahead of his or her parents, cognitively and coping-wise and have expectations for themselves not understood or shared by parents.

In those situations, when both parents and adolescents have attained the same cognitive stage, the parents often cannot accept the adolescent's newly attained cognitive gains. They feel frightened, angry, frustrated, in observing and living with their adolescent's new experimentation, which usually extends from thoughts and words to experimental acts which may jeopardize the physical condition and the safety of the adolescent.

The case vignettes given by Dr. Berlin nicely illustrate his points about mutual destructive and constructive interaction of family members around a chronically ill child. It is particularly pleasing to hear about the smooth employment of couples' therapy and family therapy with Perry, the nine year old asthmatic boy. Perry had many strikes against him from early on: being unwanted, colicky, sickly, thin, whiney, more or less a pest to everybody at home. It is notable that his asthma did not begin until the first grade, until we hear that after six months of parental therapy, the parents did recall Perry's asthma-like attacks when he was a toddler.

Dr. Berlin's play therapy with Perry should not be under-estimated. His ability to help Perry slowly express anger as well as fright about being angry represents a tour de force. After five months of combined therapies, the asthma condition began to subside. It is interesting to hear about the family meetings, giving the mother the task of helping Perry with math assignments. Many of us would not have done that because we wanted to disentangle the ambivalent relationship between mother and Perry. As expected, Perry did develop asthma attacks while studying with the mother. It could be shown to the two of them how Perry's wheezing began as the mother became impatient with Perry. The sister, Anne, was able to help the mother to listen to the wheezing, and to administer to Perry. In this way the mother became "a good mother." The family sessions also brought Anne, described as a normal blossoming adolescent girl, into the picture. Her concerns about normal adolescent sexual issues brought the parents' sexual shyness into focus. It was delightful to hear about how The Joys of Sex led the parents to a mountain cabin for a rejuvenating weekend of sensual pleasure. Indeed these seven months of family therapy, couple therapy, and a shorter time of Perry's individual therapy, were well spent by everyone involved. It illustrates how skillful inter-mingling of psychotherapeutic techniques may provide higher consumer satisfaction at a relatively low cost.

The case of the fifteen year old boy Steve, with colitis, focuses upon helping the patient and his family with Steve's many years of pent-up hostility, depression, and "feelings of being unloved." The staff and the parents were helped to understand what

was behind Steve's festering, noisy hostility. Each family member
was given tasks in helping this patient; the tasks were skillfully
arranged to cover both the present dysphoric feelings and past
conflicts, particularly related to the death of his mother when he
was five years old. The father became a therapeutic ally (or co-
therapist) in letting Steve know how he (the father) had felt during
his mother's illness and death. This is an example of the parent
providing meaningful interpretations to his child, suggesting a set
of cognitive and emotional images to the child about father's early
feelings which allowed the son to more freely express his feelings
in the present, and recall past feelings.

After five months, Steve was psychologically in markedly better
shape and was "essentially asymptomatic for colitis." However, we
do know the increased risk for colon cancer in patients with a
long history of ulcerative colitis. The long term outcome of
Steve's illness may require a colostomy of some kind.

In listening to Dr. Berlin's paper, with his refreshing examples
of family therapeutic techniques combined with individual interventions, we may wonder how we were able to handle similar patient
situations in the sixties. We have come a long way from the claims
of the 50s and 60s of individual psychoanalytic approaches curing
all kinds of childhood psychosomatic illnesses, with only minimal
involvement of the child's primary support system, the family. If
some of those early studies were true in terms of sustained follow-
up success, these individual therapeutic endeavors were long and
expensive and often left the healthy family members in limbo, if
not in psychological pain. Family treatment approches to the
problems of a physically ill child are here to say.

WHEN DO FAMILIES DEVELOP INSIGHT?   GENERAL DISCUSSION

Dr. Richard Oberfield: Audience Member--Child Psychiatrist

    I have a question for Dr. Berlin. In the two family vignettes,
you described working in an insight oriented way with both families
after what I felt was some initial resistance. How would you
proceed with a family where you get much more resistance to looking
in any insight oriented way to the problems? Does task assignment
play a role in that?

Dr. Berlin

    The model actually began with an experimental effort to deal
with disorganized families. In fact, what does occur is that insight
occurs after the tasks themselves are being worked on. There is
an interaction between those tasks which alter the feelings of the
individuals towards each other and their effectiveness in addressing
the tasks. Some "ah ha!" phenomena occur during family therapy.
With disorganized families, the intellectual aspect of insight was
almost never noted. The change in behavior is very clear, although
they do not come up with any great ideas about why the behaviors
are different. However, in fact, they do behave differently with
each other as they go through some of these tasks. We are always
asked, "How do you find out what task to ask about or to define?"
It is always amazing to find out that the tasks really ultimately
do emerge from the family. One has to begin with what seems to be
a reasonable task, and make sure the family agrees that it is
reasonable. Then, as they try to do it and you examine what the
obstacles are to doing it, they begin to come up with better tasks.

Dr. Richard Oberfield

    As a corollary, have you ever met a family where you came up
against massive resistance in relation to doing any task?

Dr. Berlin

    Yes! We have never been successful either with families where
the parents are psychotic or where the parents are impulse ridden

33

and very acting out individuals. We have never been able to work
effectively with those families.

Dr. Luis Najarian: Audience Member--Child Psychiatrist

Those early ideas about intensive psychoanalytic work with
children were developed here at Downstate many years ago by Melita
Sperling. One of the goals was to change the child in order to
help the somatic illness. More recently, we are working with the
families, as you indicated. When working with a gastroenterologist
where there are many severe cases of inflammatory bowel disease,
Crohn's disease, colitis, and ulcerative colitis, I am impressed
with the degree of varying psychopathology in the families. We
work with the families and often the somatic illness is not changed.
I am curious to know what your therapeutic success has been on
changes in bowel disease. Namely, how sick do they remain? You
try to save the kid's colon, but many times these kids go to surgery
anyway. They have significant pathology in the intestine. What
changes have you noticed in the bowel disease?

Dr. Berlin

My experience is limited to one patient and so I really can't
answer. Perhaps Dr. Mattsson can?

Dr. Mattsson

I really appreciate Dr. Berlin's honesty. You are always
honest. This is one of the few areas where I get a little up
tight, because there are no large random studies of inflammatory
bowel diseased children, adolescents and adults who were treated
with or without psychotherapy. Maybe its partly my Scandanavian
and European background, but I take a much more dim view of the
long term prognosis. This view applies even in a situation like
Steve's, where you have years of no pathology and the mucosa looks
good. I would speculate that if you follow a series of patients
for 10, 15, or 20 years, they are going to come down with polyps
or cancer at a higher rate than controls. Unfortunately, I cannot
refer to any studies. But I think we, as psychiatrists, have to
be extremely careful about claiming success. George Engel, M. D.
never made claims of long term bowel "cures" and he probably has
had more experience than anyone else in this country with ulcerative
colitis patients.

Dr. Christ

Dr. Berlin's presentation highlights the need to clarify the
relationship of two variables: physical illness and psychiatric
disturbance. One interaction is: emotionally healthy individuals
who react emotionally to severe physical illness; another is where

family members are emotionally disturbed and react to a severe
physical illness; a third, perhaps more common than the second,
where the interaction of long standing emotional illness with
severe physical illness results in a new level of physical emotional
dysfunction. All three of these need also to be separated from
those physical illnesses that are etiologically the result of the
emotional illness, not just where the physical illness is exacer-
bated by the emotional illness or the emotional reaction to the
physical illness. In light of our growing understanding about
the principle of equifinality, even the improvement or cure of an
ill individual by a specific medical or psychiatric intervention
cannot alone be used to prove a specific etiology.

EARLY INTERVENTIONS FOR FAMILIES WITH CHRONICALLY ILL CHILDREN

David M. Kaplan, Ph.D.

Stanford University School of Medicine

Palo Alto, California

The initial response of the family to the diagnosis of a chronic disease is the focus of this presentation because the origins of many of the long term psychosocial problems associated with chronic disease can be traced to this early phase. For the same reason, early interventions designed to deal with these problems at their inception are critically important.

Anyone who has had experience with serious childhood illness in families knows that the human problems generated by such illnesses are severe and often overwhelming. Living with chronically ill children not only disrupts families profoundly while the child is alive, but the survivors bear the scars of the illness experience long afterward. The following excerpt from a letter written by a parent who lost a child from cancer describes the impact of this disease:

> My wife and I lost our ten-year-old daughter to leukemia in 1970. My wife appears to have borne up well under and through the whole thing despite the pain and sorrow during the one year Susan lived from the date of diagnosis, that is, except for the fact that she had a miscarriage of the child she was carrying.

> In addition to that tribulation, I was involved in an auto accident a few months after the diagnosis. While I was still in the recovery stages, my daughter died. My mother, who was already ill, suffered a depression and had to be hospitalized.

> My youngest daughter, only three, had what I

consider a startling reaction to her older sister's death.
She wouldn't eat certain foods until her mother first
"tested" them for safety. She wouldn't touch anything
on the floor for fear of germs; and she would walk
around and not step on anything out of the ordinary. She
was only three years old, yet she questioned us constantly
about leukemia. She continues to have emotional problems
which I am unable to intelligently articulate. I still
lay awake nights thinking about her and have fits of
depression which are obvious around the holidays. My
wife and I have ulcers as a result of the one year of
waiting and watching--nothing serious.

The most peculiar thing of all is that I always
felt that as more time passed the after-effects would
gradually lessen and go away. It has been four years and
the experience is still vivid and unreal.

Other commonly observed difficulties in families with chronically ill children include:

1)   serious marital problems that often lead to divorce.
2)   parent-child relationships including well siblings that
     are aggravated by euphemistic and inaccurate communica-
     tions about the disease and its prognosis.
3)   the premature disengagement of the family from the ill
     child leading to its abandonment in hospital.
4)   unresolved grief problems that continue for years among
     survivors.
5)   "flights of activity" occur during the child's illness that
     add to the stress load in the family and waste precious
     energy and resources, e.g., pregnancies, moving to new
     communities, divorces, remarriages, etc.

Unfortunately, these problems are the rule rather than the
exception. In the early 70s, Stanford Medical Center surveyed
families with a leukemic child and found that only 15% of them
managed to survive the illness experience without serious damage to
family integrity or to individual members. Of the many problems
reported by the study families, 80% were not in existence prior to
the diagnosis of leukemia (Kaplan, 1976).

While professional interest and concern for families with
chronically ill children has been growing and more attention is being
paid to their psychosocial problems, the question of whether current
efforts to help are effective remains a moot point. My own con-
viction is that much of current clinical activity with the psychosocial problems generated by chronic physical disease consists
largely of "humpty dumpty" work. By the time treatment is instituted,

family problems are often as overwhelming to health professionals as they are to the families. The professional finds himself confronted with the impossible task of trying to put broken eggs together again.

What can we do to be more effective in helping families with seriously ill children? We can be more effective if we are willing to alter radically our approach to families with chronically ill children. Fortunately, we have the experience of others to draw upon who have successfully resolved similar problems.

RAPID INTERVENTION

During the early phases of World War II and the Korean Conflict, those soldiers who suffered psychological decompensation in combat were conceived of as patients with psychiatric diseases, and treated for neuroses and psychoses, without seriously considering the role of combat stress in these breakdowns. Those soldiers who decompensated were sent to rear echelon hospitals for traditional psychiatric treatment of chronic mental disorders. By and large, this treatment proved ineffective; the majority of these casualties did not return to their military units. They were evacuated to stateside hospitals and, eventually, discharged from service as psychiatric casualties (Glass, 1954).

Largely as a result of these early treatment failures in both wars, the subsequent treatment of combat fatigue was altered significantly. Casualties were removed from combat but kept geographically close to their units. They continued to wear their uniforms, were given hot food and a brief period of sustained rest. Many of these soldiers returned quickly to their units and functioned effectively again. Those who needed additional treatment were sent, briefly, to nearby station hospitals where, with the help of medication, they abreacted painful combat experiences. Once again, many of these soldiers returned to their units to perform effectively (Glass, 1953).

Successful results have also been achieved with individuals who decompensate under peacetime conditions (Querido, 1956; Carse, 1958; Greenblatt, 1963). Emergency treatment, which conceives of decompensation as a result of the interaction between individuals and stressful environments and not simply as an expression of a chronic emotional disorder, has proven capable of recompensating and restoring patients rapidly to useful functioning again. In Colorado, Kal Flomenhaft and I participated in an outpatient program that avoided the hospitalization of decompensated patients while it restored them rapidly to customary levels of social functioning in over 90% of the demonstration cases. The Colorado project depended heavily on brief but intensive interventions with patient families (Langsley and Kaplan, 1968).

The failure to restore casualties rapidly to useful functioning by treating chronic emotional disorders, and the success achieved by stress-oriented, brief intervention suggests the existence of an intervening variable. This variable is a unique form of psychosocial disorder that is as distinct from chronic mental disorders as the acute infectious disorders are from chronic physical diseases. There is growing evidence to support the idea of such a category of psychosocial disorders that require a distinct form of treatment as well (Kaplan, 1973, 1976, 1979; Holland, 1974).

DIAGNOSIS OF CHRONIC CHILDHOOD ILLNESS

The diagnosis of chronic childhood illness is an example of an event that heralds the end of an established pattern of family living without illness. But a family does not move tranquilly from an established pattern of wellness to a new long term state of living with chronic illness. The diagnosis precipitates a brief period of acute disturbance for all members of the family while they struggle, individually and collectively, to come to terms with the new and unwelcome reality of chronic illness.

After a brief struggle during which critical decisions are made, a new and perservering pattern of living emerges. The new living pattern may be an adaptive response which is realistically attuned to the harsh requirements of chronic illness; or the pattern may be maladaptive which ignores the meaning of chronic illness and the changes required to live realistically with it. The health professional interceding on behalf of individuals and families who are confronted with chronic disease must understand the special nature of the disorders of change that accompany these illnesses and the unique early interventions that they require. The treatment of neurosis in families suddenly confronted with chronic disease is largely irrelevant to the critical brief struggle that immediately follows the physical diagnosis.

A period of transition is not a calm or happy experience. It is a time of turmoil and suffering in which the individual reluctantly gives up a familiar and valued pattern of living while he struggles to come to terms with unwanted problems inherent in a new way of life. A transitional period is brief because the disturbance is precipitated by change sets in motion forces whose goal is to regain an equilibrium as free from the turmoil and dysfunction of crisis as possible. In this sense, transitional conditions are self-correcting, but while self-correction brings an end to the period of heightened distress, it does not necessarily mean that the new equilibrium is a good one for the long haul or that it will leave the individual free of new problems.

Acute infectious diseases are also self-correcting processes

but whether or not one emerges from them without long term damage
is another matter. The individual who survives polio may or may not
be permanently disabled. Outcome depends upon how well the physio-
logic struggle for mastery over disease has been waged. Outcome
in acute psychosocial situations also depends upon the success or
failure of the individual's struggle to master change.

During these brief transitional periods, the individual takes
the initial steps toward fashioning a new way of life in accord with
his perception of what is demanded of him by change. If his assessment is realistic, and if he can make those changes that fit his
altered circumstances, then the individual has made a good beginning
toward achieving a new and viable pattern of living. However, if he
misreads the meaning of the change that has been visited upon him
and if he fails to make sound problem-solving decisions at the outset,
for whatever reasons, he is unlikely to achieve a living pattern free
of major new problems that are apt to persist for long periods of
time.

DISORDERS OF CHANGE

The idea that transitions precipitate acute reactions is well
known; what is less well understood is the nature of these disturbances and the potentially negative consequences that follow them
when they are left unattended. I refer to these acute psychosocial
disturbances as "disorders of change." This classification constitutes a further development of crisis theory.

Disorders of change involve problem-solving struggles in which
successful outcome is linked to the resolution of common, empirically
determined coping tasks that are specific to each change. The problem-solving process involves cognitive and decision-making components as well as emotional aspects. The nature of the problem-solving
effort is reflected in the decisions that are made to solve the
problems posed by each change. These decisions are the distillates
of the coping struggle which permit us to evaluate the adequacy
of individual problem-solving efforts soon after a change occurs
Kaplan and Grandstaff, 1979).

Outcome is associated with "normal" and "morbid" courses of
response that are observable very soon after a change occurs.
Diagnosis in these disorders involves determining the adaptive or
maladaptive course of response the individual manifests in each
case situation. Individual treatment is reserved largely for maladaptive responses, i.e., for those who are unable to resolve the
coping tasks effectively and quickly. The treatment goal is to help
the individual replace ineffective problem-solving methods with
effective ones to achieve good outcome. Outcome is measured by
specific criteria that are also empirically determined. The indi-

vidual struggle in these disturbances is profoundly influenced by
current relationships and by impinging social systems (Kaplan and
Grandstaff, 1979; Kaplan and Mason, 1960).

Why is it so important to pay prompt attention to disorders
of change during their brief tenure? This question is not raised
in relation to acute infectious disorders because we recognize that
these diseases can kill or maim their victims if not quickly treated.
Unfortunately, we don't generally recognize that disorders of change
also have the capacity to cause serious harm if they do not receive
prompt treatment.

Part of the apathy toward acute psychosocial disorders is
accounted for by the fact that the damage that they cause is not
readily apparent as it is following polio. For example, women after
the diagnosis of breast cancer report a persistant diminution in
sexual activity and satisfaction; while they and their partners have
concern about these changes in their relations, this problem is
not visible to the casual observer.

During disorders of change, critical decisions have to be made
that have far reaching and often irreversible consequences. These
decisions are made in an atmosphere of high anxiety which lessens
the potential for sound decision-making. In addition, people in
crisis rarely have access to information that would facilitate good
decision-making. I. James and L. Mann (1977) point out that during
crisis, people who are faced with major personal decisions do not
get second opinions from physicians or lawyers. Consequently, they
frequently make decisions that lead to miscalculation, wishful
thinking and disillusionment. For example, after a spouse's death,
survivors often give up networks of friends and important services
in home communities to move to distant communities close to relatives.
Such moves often fail to meet expectations, leaving these migrants
without compensating relatives and supports. Retirees have similar
experiences. Yet we have no way of routinely warning people about
the risks involved in such moves. Mothers of children newly diagnosed with cancer, frequently plan to become pregnant soon again
without any awareness of the complications that accompany the conflicting needs of newborn infants and dying children. Patients and
their families are typically unaware of the choices that are possible
today and need to be made during the treatment of many forms of
cancer, e.g., osteogenic sarcoma and breast cancer.

Until quite recently, treatment choices were not possible, but
today, there are options, and some surgeons encourage their patients
to participate in making treatment decisions. Other surgeons continue to make decisions for their patients who acquiesce. It is
also clear that patients and families who participate in treatment
decisions have better psychosocial outcomes (Janis and Mann, 1977).

With a disorder of change, all interventions require a basic knowledge of what is involved in successful individual adaptation to each change. This knowledge is the keystone on which all forms of intervention in disorders of change is built. Each change poses empirically identifiable, common, individual coping tasks as well as specific behaviors that are effective in resolving those tasks. For example, E. Lindemann (1944) identified the critical task for a survivor following the death of a loved person to be freeing oneself, psychologically, from bondage to the deceased. This task is accomplished through "grief work"--the process of mourning that eventually frees the survivor and allows him to resume a meaningful and satisfying life without the deceased.

The successful resolution of stress coping tasks is a complicated process and the individual struggle to accomplish these tasks is fraught with hazards that can interfere with successful task resolution. The goal of all interventions in disorders of change is to help the individual resolve coping tasks successfully and quickly in order to achieve a healthy outcome, free of complications, much as the physician treats an infectious disease to insure healthy outcome.

Because the struggle to come to terms with changing circumstances does not occur in a vacuum, but in a social context which strongly influences the individual outcome, interventions must take diverse forms. Some interventions are directed toward the patient, others toward persons in his environment, still others toward social systems whose personnel and policies influence the coping struggle.

PSYCHOSOCIAL CONSEQUENCES OF CHILDHOOD LEUKEMIA

In order to demonstrate a strategy of multiple interventions designed to deal with the psychosocial consequences of a disease soon after the diagnosis is made, the disorder of change precipitated by the diagnosis of leukemia in a child and the responses of individuals and families to this experience will be described. A major psychological task for the individual and family posed by the diagnosis of leukemia is to recognize, as soon as possible, the essential nature of this illness. Today, leukemia, like many other forms of cancer, is a serious, chronic disorder involving exacerbations and remissions following treatment. Leukemia, for many patients, is ultimately a fatal disease. While long term survival is more likely under current treatment, it is dangerous for the patient and family to assume that leukemia is curable. The belief in a cure fosters a false sense of security and a relaxation of the vigilant attitude needed to detect signs of recurrence. Childhood leukemia still recurs in 50% of all cases within the first five years. In addition to realizing that leukemia is a chronic, recurring disease, it is important also to come to terms with the probability of ultimate fatality from this illness. Those who are able to face this eventuality, contrary to popular belief, do not dwell morbidly on this fact, but pick up their lives to make the most of the time they have left.

Recognizing the existence of a chronic disease is cause enough for grieving. The loss of one's good health is obviously something to mourn over--for both immediate and long term consequences. Chronic childhood illnesses decisively limit many desirable activities and preclude the achievement of cherished future goals. Moreover, the impact of chronic disease is not limited to the ill child, but is shared by all members of the family as well. Grieving is a natural and healthy response to the realities posed by chronic illness. It is a reaction that all members should experience, and the sooner grieving takes place, the better. One pays a high price for any substantial delay. Some families facilitate the grieving process for their members, while others set up obstacles to its accomplishment (Kaplan, 1973).

Those individuals and families who do not rapidly achieve an accurate cognitive grasp of what leukemia portends, who, for whatever reasons, are not free to grieve over its implications, will not be able to make those accommodations that are necessary to live with cancer without being totally overwhelmed by this experience. For many patients and families, living with cancer means surviving under siege conditions. In order to make those accommodations in family organization required by a siege, the accomplishment of the tasks outlined above is a prerequisite.

FAMILY MEDIATION

Just as a military siege necessitates the disciplined control of limited resources, the assumption of new and onerous responsibilities and the acceptance of undesired limitations, chronic illness also means giving up, for the duration or forever, valued goals such as buying a car or a home, taking extended vacations, seeing children through college, marriage, having grandchildren, etc.

Surveys of families with leukemic children who were without effective outside intervention, indicate that the accomplishment of the tasks described above is rarely achieved in early or later stages of the illness. We also learned that it is very difficult to play "catch up" in coming to terms with a chronic illness. If a family does not get off on the right foot, the passage of time only reinforces the poor coping decisions that were made at the outset (Kaplan, 1973).

It is important for effective intervention to take place in the earliest phases of individual and family responses to chronic illness when it becomes evident that coping efforts are not adaptive

and family members are headed for trouble. Denying the diagnosis,
attempting to carry out family affairs on a "business as usual" basis,
suppressing or inhibiting expressions of grief, searching for a
miracle cure, and discrepant parental reactions to the illness
are all issues which require immediate intervention.

When the individual family member experiences stress, the family
serves as the social system that attempts to mediate stress for its
members. The family seeks to provide those conditions that facilitate individual coping efforts. The two processes--individual coping
and family mediation--are separate phenomena even though they occur
simultaneously and may seem to be identical processes. Unlike other
systems, the family is unique in that it assumes a continuous
responsibility for mediating stress situations for its members.

When the family fulfills its mediating function well, it
strengthens individual members immensely in their coping struggle.
When the family fails to mediate stress effectively, it creates
obstacles for its members, weakens its own mediating capacity, and
possibly jeopardizes the family's continued existence. It is very
important during and after the initial crisis to protect the family
by providing interventions and services that are needed to survive
chronic stress conditions. Single parent families and those in
which parents disagree over the meaning and handling of cancer are
examples of special risk groups.

A family atmosphere of free discussion is necessary to prepare
each member for living with cancer. No one gains from attempts to
hide from unpleasant facts, although many families refuse to face
cancer and its implications for unconscionably long periods of time
after the diagnosis is made known. Effective family mediation is
also evident in the free expression of grief that follows the
diagnosis. Mutual consolation of family members is also a part of
healthy family grief reactions. Families have an obligation to
reassure the ill child that he will not be abandoned when the going
gets rough. Even very young children with cancer can sense abandonment when it is present.

Families must also be helped to maintain a balance between the
needs of the sick child and those of its well members. Some child
oncology units demand that one parent give first priority to meeting
the patient's needs even if that means seriously neglecting the rest
of the family. Other cancer units expect families to agree to the
patient's continuous participation in new treatment protocols as
long as he lives, irrespective of the quality of life. Medical
expectations of the patient and family should be subject to systematic review to protect individual and family interests.

HEALTH PROFESSIONALS

Most of the recommendations made here for the family, apply to health professionals as well. Just as the psychosocial fate of children depends heavily upon adaptive parental behavior, so are families dependent upon the constructive behavior of health professionals and health care systems to promote and support sound family mediation in disorders of change.

Intervention in these acute disorders should not be narrowly conceived or restricted to the clinical treatment of the individual who fails to cope well and who is in danger of suffering the consequences of poor outcome. Such treatment is only one aspect of a comprehensive strategy of intervention for disorders of change. Because the essential coping process in these disorders involves individual problem-solving, much can be done to enhance independent coping without resorting to clinical treatment. Direct treatment will always be limited by the large number of acute stress problems and the small number of personnel available to treat them. Independent problem-solving can be promoted by making as much information as possible available to those under acute stress. Patients and families need to be fully informed about disorders of change, about what is involved in effective problem-solving, about family mediation, and the critical decisions that have to be made. And this information has to be gotten to people early enough to be of benefit in the brief period of acute struggle.

Knowledge of effective coping with cancer makes possible yet another form of intervention, i.e., systems modification whose aim is to reduce the impact of unavoidable stress by modifying the social systems which influence individual coping. Where illness is concerned, system modification includes the practices of health care personnel and the policies of hospitals, clinics, and medical practitioners. System modification takes two forms: changing established practices and policies that hinder individual coping; and, secondly, instituting practices and policies that do not exist but which serve to support independent coping efforts. For example, many well-meaning surgeons who reassure their patients that they "got all the cancer" in order to bolster the hope of patients and their families are unwittingly encouraging them to forget about the continuing need for routine medical follow-up and self examination. This announcement promotes false hope that turns into distrust and resentment when cures do not materialize.

A major effort must be made to change the view of health care personnel toward the role of the patient and family in the treatment of cancer. A "good" patient is, far too commonly, assumed to be the docile, compliant child or adolescent who accepts recommendations from team members without question, without protest, and with gratitude. It is certainly easier to manage such passive patients

but the price for this compliance is paid for by both sides. The
health team risks losing the confidence and trust of the child and
family, while the patient may fail to achieve the psychosocial recovery he is capable of.

It is essential to recognize that individuals and families cope
best when they have accurate information about the illness they must
deal with. Unfortunately, many health professionals assume that the
truth, harsh as it may be, is not something most people can deal with
and, therefore, questions about prognosis and the effects of treatment go unanswered or are sugar coated. Parents are often given
mixed messages about the implications of the diagnosis of leukemia--
yes, it is a serious disease but it is curable or will be with
anticipated research breakthroughs. How is a family to respond to
this message? Most people can manage good news easily but bad news
must be stated unambiguously. Preparations for harsh realities
will not be made unless they are perceived as real probabilities.
Holding out hope is important as long as we do not promote false
hopes. With leukemia, the hope for good and long remissions is
realistic, but the hope for a cure can divert families from reality.
Any diversion from reality is anathema to adaptive coping and constructive mediation.

Other issues for which the medical care system should be monitored include a tendency on the part of health personnel to withdraw
from patient and family when treatment of the disease fails; a
corollary tendency is to refer "difficult" and terminally ill
patients to psychiatrists. Unfortunately, a large number of patients
referred to psychiatry because they present management problems,
assume that they are mentally as well as physically ill. Most
patients want all aspects of their care to come from the unit that
is treating their cancer. They resent their care being fractured
among different specialists. Clearly, the education of health team
members in acute stress problems is as important as the education of
the public.

While intervention is important during the initial crisis
following diagnosis, families with chronically ill children need
a good deal of help over the long haul as well. Providing emotional
support through sympathetic and knowledgeable health teams, through
peer support groups, and from extended families is very important.
So is the provision of income to pay for living and medical costs,
for rest and recreation, for baby sitting and housekeeping services
for those families that do not have the resources for these services.

CONCLUSION

The family is the crucial social system for member stress
mediation. It is the only unit that assumes this responsibility on

an ongoing basis. It must be sustained to perform this vital
function. When the family fails to fulfill this role, its members
suffer grievously and so does the community which is forced to
substitute for the family at great cost and without any mechanisms
that approach the effectiveness of this unique human organization.

REFERENCES

Carse, J., Panton, N. E., and Watt, A. A District Mental Health
    Service: The Worthing Experiment. Lancet, January 4, 1958,
    39-42.
Glass, A. J. Psychotherapy in the Combat Zone. American Journal
    of Psychiatry, 110:10, 728, 1954.
Glass, A. J. Psychiatry in the Korean Campaign: A Historical
    Review. U. S. Armed Forces Medical Journal, 4:1563-1585, 1953.
Greenblatt, M. The Prevention of Hospitalization: Treatment without
    Admission for Psychiatric Patients. New York: Grune and
    Stratton, 1963.
Holland, J., Kaplan, D. M., and Davies, S. Interschool Transfers:
    A Mental Health Challenge. Journal of School Health, XLIV:2,
    74-79, February, 1974.
Janis, I., and Mann, L. Decision Making: A Psychological Analysis
    of Conflict, Choice and Commitment, New York: Free Press,
    1977.
Kaplan, D. M., Grobstein, R., and Smith, A. Predicting the Impact
    of Severe Illness in Families. Health and Social Work, 1:3,
    August, 1976.
Kaplan, D. M., Smith, A., Grobstein, R., and Fischmann, S. Family
    Mediation of Stress, Social Work, 60-69, July, 1973.
Kaplan, D. M., Grandstaff, N. A Problem Solving Approach to Terminal
    Illness for the Family and Physician. In C. Garfield (Ed.)
    Stress and Survival, New York: Mosby Company, 343-352, 1979.
Kaplan, D. M. and Grandstaff, N. Early Case Findings and Psycho-
    social Interventions for Problem Coping Families with Breast
    Cancer. Macomber Award B-172, American Cancer Society,
    California Division, San Francisco, 1979.
Kaplan, D. M. and Mason, E. Maternal Reactions to Premature Birth
    Viewed as an Acute Emotional Disorder. American Journal of
    Orthopsychiatry, 30(30), 539-547, July, 1960.
Langsley, D. and Kaplan, D. M. The Treatment of Families in Crisis.
    New York: Grune and Stratton, 1968.
Lindemann, E. Symptomatology and Management of Acute Grief. Amer-
    ican Journal of Psychiatry, 101:2, 141-148, 1944.
Querido, A. Early Diagnosis and Treatment Services. Elements
    of a Community Mental Health Program. New York: Milbank
    Memorial Fund, 1956.

STRUGGLING FOR SURVIVAL: DISCUSSION OF DR. KAPLAN'S PAPER

H. Paul Gabriel, M.D.

New York University Medical Center

New York, New York

This is a wide-ranging analysis of the factors that affect
children and their families when faced with overwhelming chronic
disease. The author quite rightly compares those issues, both intrafamilial and extrafamilial, with the phenomena observed in combat,
for it seems to this discussant that, indeed, these families are
embroiled in overwhelming struggles for survival. Certainly, there
is no doubt that they are swept into a crisis atmosphere that is
both the result of their disease and externally imposed by the
institutions which are geared to dealing with the overwhelming
biological threat to the organism.

There is no question that the rapidity and intensity of these
interventions causes a "crisis of change" and can result in disorders
of change. I could not agree more with the proposition that early
and effective interventions would be the most effective way to cope
with the potential of maladaptive adjustment. Unfortunately, I also
must agree that the systems in which we work present all of us with
significant problems in providing the best and most comprehensive
approach to these major family crises. The issues that the author
raises must be considered indeed pressing and problematical in an
age of retrenchment and diminishing rather than increasing support
systems.

As with any provocative presentation, many questions come to
mind that are difficult to answer and represent a challenge to all
of us who work in this field. First, as in the case of the Coconut
Grove disaster mentioned by Dr. Kaplan, and perhaps the tragedy at
Buffalo Creek, one is not entirely sure that even the best of interventions can mitigate completely the potential of losing one's child.
Furthermore, one must say that people bring to war or to catastrophe

49

a whole host of prior developmental and life experiences that have
shaped their personalities and family organizations for many years
before they face their child's illness. All of us, I think, are
cognizant of and clearly respect both the individual's and family's
need for whatever defensive systems it has when dealing with the
onslaught of life-threatening illness in one of the members of the
family. Indeed, the author quite accurately points out that sometimes premature grief and premature working through or mourning
can lead to isolation of the child, both by staffs and occasionally
by families who have completed the work of separation. I believe
that it was at the National Institute of Mental Health that
Friedman and Hamburg (1963) wrote a paper on the "Dying Child
Syndrome" which indicated that parents who had been informed that
their child was dying (usually after an automobile accident) prematurely separated from the child. When the child survived, problem
sequelae flowed from the fact that the family had already completed
the work of separation. It is very difficult in this day of changing
percentages of survival to predict accurately the outcome of life-
threatening chronic disease. When I started in this work 15 years
ago, the problem was relatively simple: we helped the families deal
with the death of their child, since in 90% of cases of malignant
tumors, for example, death was inevitable. Now, there is no such
thing as inevitable in pediatrics, except by the gun, the knife, or
the car. This makes the job of the physician and the helping professional far more complicated and problematical. There are, in
fact, even times when one wonders whether one should support denial
for a while in the face of rapidly changing approaches. Nonetheless,
I do wholeheartedly agree that thoughtfulness, honesty, and direct
early dealing with the families around the potential severity of
the disease has very much to recommend it. The concept of early
intervention is one which we must all make major efforts to
implement and maintain as well as educating our medical colleagues
to the need to be more effective in their management of these
serious family crises. There is no doubt that these families are
waging a long and hard war, sometimes for more than two or three
years before they can know the outcome, and while one is appalled
by the rapidly accumulating statistics of family disintegration in
the face of these onslaughts, it is, sad to say, not entirely unex-
prected. As the author indicates, we must all be cognizant of the
potential dangers to the families and do our utmost to moderate
and mitigate maladaptive responses.

REFERENCES

Friedman, S. B., Chodoff, P., Mason, J. W., and Hamburg, D. A.
    Dying Child Syndrome. Journal of Pediatrics, 32, 610-625, 1963.

TREATMENT OF THE FAMILY'S DENIAL OF A DYING CHILD: GENERAL DIS-

CUSSION

Dr. Kaplan

I was reminded by Dr. Gabriel's comments about anticipatory grief, which may be done too well too early. Erich Lindeman described this phenomenon at the end of World War II when there were many women whose husbands were in combat. They simply found it too difficult to live with the idea that any day a telegram could come saying, "Your husband is missing in action." Indeed, they went through this process of detaching themselves from their husbands. When the husbands came home, there was nothing left of the marriage and the families broke up. I don't mean to suggest that the history of the family and of the individual do not count. History does count. What interests me is that we cannot do a hell of a lot about the history of the individual. When we try, it takes years and years, if indeed, it's ever successful. Let us grant that that is possible. Nevertheless, the question remains: What can one do here and now? If, in fact, we see people making decisions now which they might be prevented from making, this is a strong case for getting in there quickly. Just as with the treatment of a septic sore throat, penicillin must be used quickly. If you wait until the other organs in the body like the heart valves are damaged, buckets of penicillin would not help. I want to underscore the importance of the earliest possible intervention.

The issue of denial always elicits a lot of discussion. How long does the practitioner go along with the idea that this father or this mother simply refuse to believe that their child has cancer? You have to try very hard to turn that around. If the patient lives for an indeterminate period of years, and as Dr. Gabriel points out, it's much longer now than in the past, a seige mentality develops which does not allow for making preparations unless one really has dealt with the possibility of having a terminal illness. I am arguing for the idea that at some point, early on, one must be prepared for the worst outcome. If one does that, one can then pick up and go on living. Then one is not in the position of so many families at the Stanford Medical Center who, after years and

51

years of lots and lots of evidence that the child was very seriously
ill, only reacted to the death, when the child was imminently dying
that very day. They had not made the preparations that are essential
to make.

Dr. Sargent

You both seem to be emphasizing the problem of dealing with
uncertainty. Have you developed specific techniques that you use
with families to help deal with uncertainty?

Dr. Gabriel

Based on the last couple of years of working intensively with
our oncology group, my belief is that we don't have any receipe for
working with these feelings of uncertainty. I tend now to be a
little more cautious in looking at families and respecting family
dynamics. Coming from a more psychoanalytic bias, I feel that
history is most important in dealing with families. In certain
instances, there is great importance in giving individual treatment.
I have now worked with eight patients, each one for over two years,
and it's very wearing, tremendously stressful. I need to follow
the family's feelings and deal with the dynamics as they arise.
But I just don't know what the optimum receipe is. An individual
who has lived through those experiences might possibly tell us
something. I read the scientific literature and I am not sure it
gives us a receipe. The literature just tells you **how** to survive
one way or another.

Dr. Kaplan

Probably the most important thing is to provide the family with
a respite, with the opportunity to recharge their internal battery,
and to get away from the chronic situation just as it was done
very effectively with soldiers in combat. Some families are blessed.
They have money, extended families, friends, and a whole array of
services. These families have an incalculable advantage. For those
families who don't have this advantage, I think it has to be provided.
The alternative is that they tend to become progressively dysfunctional.

Dr. Solter: Audience Member--Psychiatrist

Dr. Gabriel has almost answered my question. I wonder how
these decisions for helping the families can be made without
intensive knowledge of the pre-morbid history of the family or the
child? Many families come into a situation with a set pattern of
making decisions, distorting information that effects how we respond
to them. I am curious about how we can go about helping these

families make decisions if we don't have some knowledge of what that family was like before all of this happened?

Dr. Kaplan

Let me give you an example of what we found ourselves doing. A mother of childbearing age hears that her child is fatally ill. She is thinking, even if she is not saying it out loud, "I am going to have another baby. I am going to get pregnant right away." We would then say quite directly to these mothers, "You may be thinking that having another baby might be a way of making yourself feel better. We strongly urge you to give this lots and lots of thought before you go ahead." We explain the problems that have been observed in families who were dealing with a dying child on the one hand, and another one coming along. Obviously, this is not a happy situation.

I am not suggesting that you always succeed and break through the defenses. It is important for the adult patient to know and to be told that he has cancer. As practitioners, we cannot be responsible for what the patient is going to do with that information. However, I think it's very important for them to have that knowledge and have the right to do with it what they choose. Similarly, parents of dying children need to be given information about typical responses that can be dysfunctional.

Dr. Solter

What type of woman would decide to have another child in that situation? Why is she deciding that as opposed to another woman who would not do that? I agree with you that the information is necessary, but why does that particular woman respond that way?

Dr. Kaplan

I don't know, I really don't know. We have not explored that decision making process in the families.

Dr. Christ

Dr. Solter and Dr. Gabriel are raising a question highly pertinent to this conference: How relevant is psychodynamic exploration with families who have a seriously ill child? My own experience is that under most circumstances, it is less relevant than other approaches, such as education, support, and reality testing. Thus, almost regardless of parental psychopathology, information about the probable inadvisability of precipitous pregnancy is in the vast majority of situations many times more important and relevant than psychodynamic explorations. On the other hand, in the small number

of parents who are seriously psychiatrically disturbed, psychodynamic
exploration of the idiosyncratic meaning of the current situation
is extremely important, perhaps more so than education, support, or
reality testing.

DEATH AND CHRONIC INCAPACITY: LONG TERM FOLLOW-UP ON ADAPTIVE

STRESSES IN A FAMILY

Adolph E. Christ, M.D.

Downstate Medical Center - Kings County Hospital

Brooklyn, NY

Introduction

Medical illness is a leveler, striking people from all walks of life with diverse coping skills and abilities. Our orientation to severely stressed and distressed families needs to encompass the inherent coping skill potential of a family as well as the severity and chronicity of the coping task being faced by the family. Further, our family theories and family therapies must begin to tackle the task of providing useful insights into the treatment of psychologically normal and healthy but overwhelmingly stressed families, rather than concentrating exclusively on the treatments of the psychologically ill.

If family theory and family therapy paradigms are to be maximally useful in addressing the problems brought about by medical illness, we will need to develop treatment and assessment skills that address not only the disturbed population, such as the skewed, the schismatic, the enmeshed, the pseudomutual, but also the Toms, the Dicks, the Harrys who represent the nondisturbed segment of the population.

Medical illness strikes emotionally disturbed and emotionally healthy. The therapeutic techniques used with these populations may need to be quite different, as do the measures used to define need for such therapeutic interventions. The former, that is, the therapeutic interventions that can be used in a situation when physical illness stress is present in an emotionally disturbed family, is exemplified in Dr. Berlin's (1982) presentation. In contrast, Mrs. Christ's (1982) concept of dys-synchrony is an effort to address the problem of assessing the origins of physical illness related stress in emotionally normal families.

55

There is a singular lack of yardsticks that can be used to measure long term adequate adaptation to long term stress in a family.
As will be exemplified in the S. family, Erickson's (1953) Eight
Stages of Man can be used as a rough approximation of the developmental sequence of a family under chronic stress. Developmental
fixation, that is, the lack of movement to the next stage of development, distinguished the response of the S. family to two major
stresses: the death at age 3 of the oldest son from cancer, and the
chronic neurological incapacity of the youngest son.

Case Example

Two events figure prominently in the life of the S. family: the
death of their first son at age three, and the chronic incapacitation
of their youngest son. Mr. and Mrs. S. each come from a hard working
success oriented extended family. Both are now in their late forties, born in the United States of emigrant parents. There are a
surprisingly large number of prominent M.D.s and Ph.D.s among their
siblings and cousins. Mr. S. shares ownership of a clothing store
with his brother; Mrs. S. is a school teacher.

The oldest son of Mr. and Mrs. S. was also the first grandson on
both sides, a fact that has great significance in a Jewish family.
A brain metastasis was the first symptom of an adrenal tumor, discovered when the mother was pregnant with her second child. The pain
of the treatment, the lack of development of the toddler, and their
decision to terminate treatment and "let him go" are described in the
interview that follows.

The following excerpts are verbatim transcripts of a videotape
made expressly for this conference. This first segment includes a
discussion of the events that led to the death of their first son.
The author is interviewing Mr. and Mrs. S.

VIDEOTAPE SEGMENT I

Mrs. S.   We had brought him to the Head of Pediatrics at Memorial
           Sloan Kettering Cancer Hospital. He took a number of
           tests, some x-rays, and gave him two to five months to
           live. An operation would have been out of the question,
           he said.

Mr. S.   And he got blind almost immediately.

Mrs. S.   Then he got x-ray treatments and lost all his hair.

Mr. S.   The first notice we had of this illness was when his eyes
           bulged out.

Mrs. S.   He had a little black mark around his eyes. We did not
           know what it was. This was my first baby and we were young

parents. My family doctor was the one who came over to our house and said, he is not sure, it might not be anything, or it might be something bad. I took him to a hospital.

Dr. C.   So that was your first indication....

Mrs. S.   We took the road, and it was downhill all the way. All kinds of treatment.

Mr. S.   He had 25 transfusions.

Mrs. S.   And numerous x-ray treatments.

Mr. S.   We would take him to the hospital for a week or two, then home for a week, then back. There was a period of time....

Mrs. S.   We were devastated. My parents were hurt. My father was very, very hurt.

Dr. C.   Was your father helpful to you at all during that period?

Mrs. S.   The baby had to have a few treatments, x-ray treatments. My father wouldn't let either of us go in for the treatments; he held the baby. He insisted on holding him.

Dr. C.   I see. Why was that?

Mrs. S.   Well, we were young, and with the x-rays, etc., etc., he said he would take care of it.

Mr. S.   He had to be held under the x-ray machines. I think I went in once or twice, I don't remember.

Mrs. S.   Besides that, I was pregnant with Melvin. They would have been 11 months apart. That was terrible, I mean tears, I can't tell you. More tears, tears. Just the unhappiness of the whole thing. I really wondered; why us? What reason? There were times we felt we were being punished. I know this is not so, that there is no reality to that, but why? Just awful, awful, awful.

Mr. S.   I felt that if the pediatrician had found it in time, maybe he would have survived. He examined the abdomen, the baby regularly. I felt he should have found it before the eye bulged out.

Mrs. S.   Maybe it was something you couldn't catch in time. I don't know.

Mr. S.   It was the neurosurgeon who said "You came too late", you know.

Dr. C.   Is that what he said?

Mr. and Mrs. S.
            Yes, that's what he said.

Dr. C.   So that your feeling was maybe if you had come earlier....

Mr. S.   Yes, before the eye bulged out....

Dr. C.   I see.

Mr. S.   Before the eye bulged out, because that already showed
            that it had spread throughout the body.

Mrs. S.   It was just terrible.

Dr. C.   Families react in different ways to such illnesses. You
            mentioned that your father got involved in helping you with
            the boy.

Mrs. S.   Yes he did.

Dr. C.   How about the rest of the family? Did they help?

Mrs. S.   My younger sister was working at the time and the baby
            needed transfusions. She did get all the people in her
            office to come down and give blood for him--that was
            helpful.

    Several themes emerge: A first son with a deadly disease in a
young family; the mother pregnant with the second child before the
parents discover the first son is ill. What adaptive and maladaptive mechanisms are at play? There is some mobilization of the
extended family--the grandfather holds the baby for the radiation
therapy so the young parents are spared the possible effects of the
radiation, one sister mobilizes her co-workers to donate blood,
another finds the name of the "best" pediatric neurosurgical oncologist.

    Both parents wondered if they were being punished, although the
next immediate association was criticism and bitter complaints about
the medical staff: the family pediatrician may not have diagnosed
the illness early enough, hence the interpretation of the neurosurgeon's statement, "It is too late." Other themes not transcribed,
were discussed by the family. The family needed more factual
information, so they bought a medical book about the illness;
the boy was not always covered on the ward the way mother would have
liked; but more strongly emphasized by them, was the absence of what
both parents described as "the human element"--a sense that the
staff knew what they were experiencing. The parents sorely missed
some discussion about the human feelings they were experiencing with
any of the professional staff.

It is hard to convey in this transcript the degree of involvement evidenced by Mr. and Mrs. S. in the events surrounding the illness and death of their first son 23 years ago. The mourning of a child's death by the parents may never be as complete or as completable as other mourning. This author feels that the mourning of a son or daughter can never be completed, and that Mr. and Mrs. S's expression of emotional involvement with their dead son is within normal limits.

The parents continue to describe the impact of the events on them:

VIDEOTAPE SEGMENT II

Mrs. S.   We wanted him to know that here is a happy home. We kept him home and tried to keep him happy. He learned how to walk even if by just walking around my furniture. I still have my original bedroom set, and you can see all the teeth marks. When he was teething he would bite into the furniture. It's still there. I keep that. Why, I don't know. I just keep that. We would take him out every weekend, on Sundays, when Marvin (Mr. S.) didn't work, we would take him for a ride in the car. He liked ice cream cones. Even though he couldn't see it, he enjoyed tasting it.

Dr. C.   That was how long ago?

Mrs. S.   Just about 22 years ago. He would be 25 in two weeks.

Dr. C.   You know, as you talk about it, it feels so alive to me, it's like it happened very recently.

Mrs. S.   It's so alive to me. He is still alive to me.

Mr. S.   It doesn't seem so long ago.

Dr. C.   It doesn't?

Mr. S.   No.

Mrs. S.   I have pictures of him when he was a few months old. It's just a normal little boy with red hair, right? (Turns to husband--both are deeply moved--their eyes show tearing). Cutest little thing--and then, I don't know, how did it happen? I just don't know.

Dr. C.   The blindness was about the first stage, and then the loss of hair....

Mr. S.   Yes, that came from the x-ray treatment.

Dr. C.   Were there any other problems in the illness itself?

Mrs. S.   Well, he never really learned to talk...never really
            learned to talk. I guess the medication, or the disease,
            whatever it was, took its effect there. We hugged him
            and held him and hoped that he would say something to us...
            It was just like holding a little rag doll.

Dr. C.   Towards the end, then, you brought him back to the hospi-
            tal? Was he still receiving treatment at that point, or
            was it that something happened that made you feel that you
            had to bring him back?

Mrs. S.   No, we would bring him back for regular visits. They took
            blood tests, and they did this, and they did that.

Mr. S.   It showed up in the blood test.

Mrs. S.   Yes, so this time when we took him back, we had to leave
            him, you know, we had to keep him there. I guess maybe
            his bood level was low. They took a blood count every
            time he came, but that time he had to stay. One of the
            doctors had asked us to please stay. So I stayed with
            him.

Dr. C.   Did you know why?

Mrs. S.   I didn't want to know why, but I knew.

Dr. C.   You knew.

Mrs. S.   I knew. I didn't want to know. At the end they were
            giving him a bone marrow test. They were transplanting
            bone marrow. It was a lady doctor--I don't recollect
            her name at this moment--she was giving him this bone
            marrow test and he was trying to drink his bottle of tea
            and I knew he was suffering. I said "No more", don't give
            him anymore tests, just leave him alone. Let him go."
            They unhooked everything and they let him go. I couldn't
            take it anymore.

Dr. C.   It takes a lot of courage to be able to do that.

Mrs. S.   Sighs.

     The decision to terminate treatment on a child is for each fam-
ily one of the hardest decisions to make. Mrs. Christ (1982) described the frequency with which dys-synchrony between father and
mother can complicate the timing of their decision in psychologically normal families. We will shortly hear more about the father's
involvement.

There are risks that are taken in such a decision -- parents risk blaming themselves or each other, developing guilt, perhaps even the rationalized content for a subsequent depression. It is probable that these more maladaptive outcomes are seen in psycho-pathological individuals rather than in normal families who face horrendous stress.

The parents continue describing the sequence of events at the terminal stage of the illness. In the midst of their very touching, sad recollections, their use of humor as a normal protective device is evident.

VIDEOTAPE SEGMENT III

Mr. & Mrs. S.
            He was in such bad shape, black and blue, all colors. He was suffering.

Mrs. S.   His skin was white, you know, like mine, and with all these needles, everything is black and blue.....

Mr. S.   I guess the disease discolored his face -- all kinds of colors like a prize fighter, you know what I mean. Like he was punched in the face.

Mrs. S.   As much as I loved him, I just couldn't see him suffer anymore.

Mr. S.   True, true.

Dr. C.   Was this something you talked over together?

Mrs. S.   About letting him go?

Dr. C.   Yes.

Mrs. S.   It just came out of me. It just came out. I couldn't see him suffer another minute. It just broke me.

Dr. C.   (turning to Mr. S.)
            How about your own reaction to that?

Mrs. S.   When it was over?

Dr. C.   To your wife deciding to end the treatment.

Mr. S.   Oh, I was there.

Mrs. S.   He was there.

Dr. C.   So you were in full agreement?

Mr. S.   Oh yes.

Dr. C.   Yes, those are the really hard moments of being a parent.

Mrs. S.   They hurt. They hurt, and they hurt, over and over again,
              all through the years. On birthdays, and on special days,
              and on holidays, and even on the birthdays of the other
              children. You think of that.

Dr. C.   Hm.

Mr. & Mrs. S.
              Yes, yes.

Mr. S.   I remember saying it to myself, even though he was blind,
              I always hoped he would live.

Mrs. S.   We would take care of him. We would always be able to take
              care of him.

Mr. S.   Before the end, he had been blind for quite awhile. It
              would be easy to overcome the problems of his blindness as
              long as he could live.

Dr. C.   Ah. You would be willing to live with that.

Mr. & Mrs. S.
              Yes, yes.

Dr. C.   And do whatever was necessary?

Mr. & Mrs. S.
              Yes

Mrs. S.   Whatever we could do for him. He was ours and we loved
              him.

Dr. C.   That was when you were pregnant with your second son?

Mrs. S.   With Melvin.

Mr. S.   He was born February 1, and the first one passed away al-
              most a year and twenty days later. That was a hard year.

Mrs. S.   Very hard. Oh God, it was terrible.

Dr. C.   That first year.

Mr. S.   When Melvin was born, taking care of him. He was a baby.
              And with two babies in diapers, and one so sick, you
              know....

Mrs. S.   I was terrified. Everytime I diapered Melvin I would
           worry. I always did if there was anything wrong with him.
           We would just, you know, be afraid that the whole world
           would collapse. So that was constantly on my mind. Con-
           stantly.

Mr. S.   We had the same obstetrician and pediatrician that de-
           livered the first one, also delivered the second one. The
           pediatrician told us that when Melvin was born, they went
           over him with a fine tooth comb. You know, to check every-
           thing, and I guess they did.

Dr. C.   Obviously there was still something that you were always
           thinking about.

Mr. S.   Oh yes, it was always on our mind.

Dr. C.   Then after your second son, your daughter was how much
           younger?

Mrs. S.   She is two years younger than Melvin.

Dr. C.   So you got pregnant shortly after your first son passed
           away?

Mr. S.   Yes, a year later. We wanted a replacement.

Dr. C.   Is that what it was?

Mrs. S.   Not really. I had always wanted four children. I said at
           least half the ones my mother had. She had eight.

Dr. C.   She had eight

Mrs. S.   I figured I wanted four.

Dr. C.   (turning to Mr. S.) Did you have anything to say about
           that?

Mr. and Mrs. S.
           (Laughing) No.

Dr. C.   I see, I see. (also laughing)

Mrs. S.   (Laughing) He has nothing to say about that!

     Clearly we see sadness and mourning in this family. There con-
tinues to be sadness and grief during certain anniversaries. Mother
describes keeping the bedroom furniture with the child's teething
marks. The event has changed the course of their continued develop-
ment--the question is, whether within normal or pathological pa-

rameters? Erickson described the developmental task during this period of life as generativity versus stagnation. Father hints at the third child being a replacement, but Mother points out that their generative plan, to have four children, antedates the boy's illness, and is adhered to. The enmeshment and the maternal dominance are clear—but are they of pathological proportions? The parents, but also the pediatrician and the obstetrician, were hyperalert to the physical well being of the next child.

Had no other calamity befallen this family, I feel the altered state of the family, including that of the next children, following the death of the first son would have fallen within normal limits. There would be some danger about being over-protective with the other children, some heightened mistrust of the medical profession, an increased sense of vulnerability to extraneous events, moments of shared sadness that could enhance the closeness of the parents with each other, but otherwise, the potential for a normal loving working "generative" life are there.

But life dealt other cards to this family. Milton, the fourth child, developed asthma at 11 months of age. By age 8 his asthma was uncontrolled with all agents, including by now high doses of steroids. A year of intensive psychotherapy at age six in a university clinic for Milton clarified his infantilization by the parents. To abort attacks, one or the other parent would stay in his bedroom until he was asleep, on occasion giving him a baby bottle for comfort, or, when an attack was starting, telling him to wet the bed rather than risk getting up to go to the bathroom. We must keep in mind that as often as 2-3 times per week they rushed Milton to the local hospital for injections to control asthma attacks, and that twice he almost died, requiring being hooked up to a heart-lung machine. Here we begin to see how the previous experience with the death of the first child may have made them more vulnerable to what is, in any case, a frightening experience for parents and siblings.

The pediatric allergist recommended Milton be sent to a nationally prominant asthma research hospital in another part of the United States. Despite the "parentectomy", a procedure described as essential by that center, the steroid-dependent asthma did not improve. After being in that hospital for about six months, Milton came home for the Christmas holidays. While playing Monopoly with his older brother and sister, Milton fell unconscious. His older brother described to me: "What made me so scared was that he was stiff, his lips and fingertips were blue—I was afraid he was going to die."

The father was called at work, and within one hour Milton was at the local hospital getting emergency treatment. Whether the result of status asthmaticus, status epilepticus, or cardial arrest secondary to the intravenous medication given to control the epilepsy, he suffered a severe anoxic episode, was comatose for over 24 hours, and did not recognize his parents or remember where he

lived for several days thereafter. He was transferred to a university hospital for extensive neurological evaluations. The primary findings were a severely abnormal EEG (slow waves) and the profound memory loss. He rapidly improved, and within a month was returned to the asthma center. The parents describe a severe personality change in Milton. A further neurological assessment at the
university medical center, affiliated with the asthma center, showed
a nearly normal EEG, and no other significant neurological findings.

At the end of a full year's hospitalization, Milton came home.
He was home about one year. The parents now describe having a
severely asthmatic child who, in addition, was quite unmanageable.
The health class teacher could not tolerate his angry outbursts and
other destructive behavior, and he seemed unable to learn. He was
returned to the asthma research center for an unprecedented second
year, where he received intensive psychotherapy for severe sudden
episodic "scared" feelings, explosive angry outbursts, seclusiveness,
and by now, unwillingness to cooperate and play with other children.
None of these were problems before his unconscious episode.

At the end of that year, Milton returned home with recommendations that he and the family get relaxation therapy and that he re-

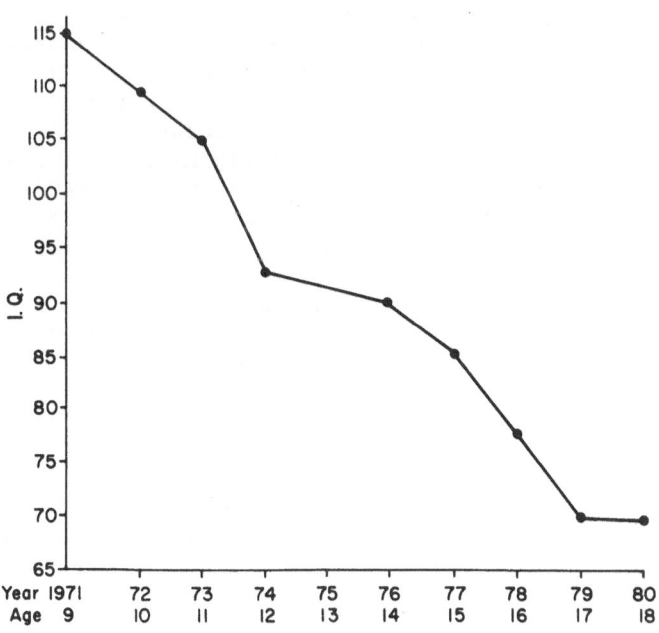

Fig. I. WISC full scale I.Q. of Milton, age 9-18 years.

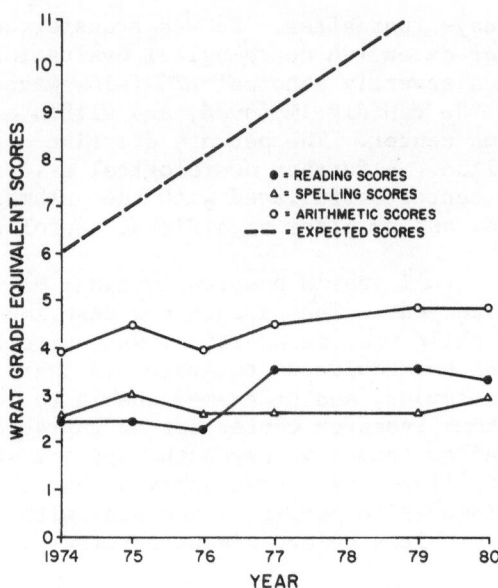

Fig. II. WRAT scores of Milton.

turn to a regular school. Two years later, the family saw me for
help in finding an appropriate school because he still was not
learning, and for some help in managing the severe emotional up-
heavals and the continuing episodic scared feelings. It rapidly
became apparent that, in addition to the severe asthma, the
"cushinoid" appearance secondary to the steroids, and the severe
fears and behavior problems, that clinically Milton had a temporal
lobe epilepsy, subsequently substantiated with sleep EEG's, and a
profound memory defect, probably secondary to the anoxic episode
that may have bilaterally injured his hypocampal structures.

     Although enrolled in an excellent special school where a great
deal of individual attention could be provided, the organic memory
problem is insurmountable. The gradually decreasing WISC scores
(see Figure I) and the unchanged WRAT scores (see Figure II) depict
the lack of cognitive development of Milton.

     Mr. and Mrs. S. next describe the stress produced on them by
the chronic incapacity of Milton. The affective tone conveyed in
the video-tape is now quite different. In discussing the first son,
there was a feeling of sadness, of shared mourning, of tenderness
and warmth. In discussing this son, there is bitterness, a sense

of hopelessness and helplessness, of anger, of depression, of helpless rage, of giving up.

    The parents have been describing Milton's behavior difficulties
and his scholastic problems. The interview now turns to an assessment of the impact of Milton's difficulties on the siblings, and the
parents' way of handling this.

VIDEOTAPE SEGMENT IV

<u>Dr. C.</u>	I was wondering about the impact of these kinds of ex- periences on parents, on brothers and sisters. Do you have any thoughts about that?
<u>Mrs. S.</u>	Sure, sure. We have a lot of thoughts about that! The first is to take those two kids out of the house--away from the problems we must go through constantly. I couldn't get Milton out of the house. I had to take care of him. We both do. So I had Melvin try for college. He won one of the Regents Scholarships and went there. I would love to keep them home. They are precious, the two of them. Wonderful kids, but I sent Melvin on his way. Much as I loved him. And when Meleta, two years later, also was a Regents....
<u>Mr. S.</u>	One year later.
<u>Mrs. S.</u>	Sorry, one year later, right she was a year ahead in school even though she was two years younger, I sent her away. The two beautiful things in our life we sent away, because I figured that was a way to solve the situation. I didn't want them to suffer, because it is suffering. There is no question about it. They would have been hurt. They couldn't bring their friends when they wanted to. They didn't know how he would treat the friends. You feel bad. It's a terrible situation. This way, Melvin went away, had four nice years, now he is in graduate school in Cali- fornia, in podiatry school--very happy. Melita found a husband in college, and she is very happy.
<u>Mr. S.</u>	(Laughing) Found a husband?
<u>Mrs. S.</u>	(Laughing) No I don't mean found, they met each other. I didn't send her for that! I didn't want her to meet any- body at 17, but all right, so some good came out of it. I still miss her very much. I miss them both very much. But I say I did the right thing. That was the right thing to do.

Dr. C.   To encourage them to leave as soon as it is practical for
          them to do so. What impact do you think it had on their
          whole development, their association with Milton?

Mrs. S.   I think terrible.

Dr. C.   In what way?

Mrs. S.   Maybe they felt that we threw them out a little bit too
          soon. Maybe they wanted to stay with us. I don't know.

Dr. C.   Once they were old enough to go to college or before that?

Mr. S.   Before that they had an obligation for him. I mean when-
          ever we wanted it. We did not go out, we hardly ever go
          out, but whenever we even wanted to go to the groceries,
          supermarket, we would leave him in charge of Milton.

Mrs. S.   Cause he could give him shots too.

Mr. S.   Shots, he could play with him, play endless games with him.

Mrs. S.   Card games.

Mr. S.   Play endless games with him, keep him occupied.

Mrs. S.   So Melvin was sort of obligated to do that and he did it.
          He never argued, but I bet he didn't want to do it all the
          time.

Dr. C.   Did he ever talk about his feeling that?

Mrs. S.   Yes. He talked about it.

Dr. C.   What did he say?

Mrs. S.   He felt...when he talked to me...I mean, I spoke to him
          many times...he felt sorry for him. He also felt sorry
          for me. Something like, "It's not fair", and I would
          say "He is my son, too. I have to take care of him,
          Melvin, don't worry about it. You will be going off to
          school. You will be on your own." And I thanked him every
          time he stayed with Milton. I felt a little relieved for
          an hour or two. And even now, when he is in California
          and we telephone, he says "When I come home, I'll stay
          with Milton for you, while you can go to the movies with
          Daddy." Even now.

Dr. C.   So he continues with that kind of feeling....

Mrs. S.   That feeling of responsibility. Melita is more sensitive.
            Well, Melvin is a sensitive boy too. Melita is very sen-
            sitive. And she is afraid to be near Milton. She fears.
            Once she was in charge of Milton, I believe it was last
            summer, and they got into a little argument. Milton is
            very argumentative, very, and he ran out of the house and
            ran away. She was so upset. She cried that it was her
            fault. Oh, she was a wreck. We finally located him, but
            she was a wreck.

Dr. C.   So there is this strong feeling of responsibility....

Mr. S.   Yes, right. They don't need it. They shouldn't have to
            have it! Kids shouldn't have this. It's not fair.

Dr. C.   Did they ever talk about the resentment of Milton?

Mr. S.   Yes, at times. They resent the attention we had to give
            Milton instead of to them.

Mrs. S.   But I think they have overcome that. I think they realize
            why. They realize why.

Dr. C.   So they would talk about it.

Mr. and Mrs. S.
            Yes, yes.

Dr. C.   That's very good.

Mrs. S.   They became very independent. They had to cook for them-
            selves. Bake. Our kids can cook and bake and clean and do
            everything for themselves.

Mr. S.   We went to the asthma center a week at a time, I think it
            was, and we left them home alone, Melita was 12 and Melvin
            was 14, and they managed very well.

Mrs. S.   My mother would just check up. She would come and see how
            they were at nights and if they needed anything, but they
            were good housekeepers. They learned how to manage, sad
            that they had to do it so young, but they did.

Now we can see clinging and some infantilization of the two
siblings--leaving home for college is not seen as a normal event,
but as an abnormal rupture. One can speculate that the death of the
first son, and the all-but-death of the fourth child was not adequately resolved to allow the normal though difficult second individuation-separation stage of development of the siblings by the
parents.

The parents are now going to explore the effect of Milton on them. They describe their depression, their alienation from the extended family, and their own stagnation.

VIDEOTAPE SEGMENT V

Dr. C.   Let me ask about the effect of all of this on you. You have had two very different experiences. One has to do with the sudden very serious illness terminating in the death of a baby. The other one has to do with a very chronic problem. By the way, the asthma seems to be much better at this point?

Mr. S.   Yes the asthma is much better.

Mrs. S.   Yes, it is a two-fold problem.

Dr. C.   But then on top of the asthma this horrendous memory defect and the behavior change. What about those two effects on you? What has this done to your lives?

Mrs. S.   Well, it has made Marvin grey on the outside, and me grey on the inside.

Dr. C.   Really?

Mr. S.   No, I think I am grey on the inside too, very grey.

Mrs. S.   I get more miserable.

Mr. S.   It's very depressing.

Mrs. S.   It's depressing, I would say....

Mr. S.   You don't know how you are going to cope with it any longer.

Mrs. S.   Because at times he is very bad. Very bad.

Mr. S.   Like yesterday, just yesterday I had to go to the Work Activity Center and pick him up. He wouldn't get on the bus. When I came there, his shirt was off. I imagined they had to hold him down, put him on the floor even, because he got so violent. He gets provoked by things that the normal person wouldn't. An incident gets started from some minute thing, like a shove, or a push, or not paying attention to him as he feels he needs, or not listening to what he is saying as he might want, or not giving him the right answer, and he is off the wall. I had to go pick him up since he wouln't get on the bus.

Dr. C.   And this is ongoing?

Mr. S.   This ongoing! It never stops.

Mrs. S.   I wish I could help Milton. Sometimes I get so angry, I
            get so mad, I figure I have got to get an answer. I've
            got to get an answer.

Mr. S.   Susan has written to everybody.

Mrs. S.   I have written to every agency. We have been to more
            doctors than you can shake a stick at. Trying, just try-
            ing.

Mr. S.   We even tried "mumbo-jumbo."

Mrs. S.   I am willing to change religion, anything that would help
            Milton.

Dr. C.   In terms of the effects of these two situations, which
            are really so hard, which do you think is the harder?

Mr. S.   (Laughing) I knew you were going to ask that!

Mrs. S.   With the first situation, you cry, then you stop crying.
            With this one, you cry and you keep on crying. I think
            we will cry forever.

Mr. S.   In my book, he can aggravate so badly that sometimes you
            wish that he would go. It's so bad. He threatens to jump
            out the window, to take the pills.

Mrs. S.   One night just about a month ago he was in one of those
            moods, and he threatened to take all the pills in the
            kitchen. He was really obnoxious. I said, "Well, if you
            think that's the right thing to do, Milton, that's what
            you have to do." And he took a whole bottle of his pills.
            Then he stood in the kitchen, looking at me, and asked,
            "What do you think is going to happen to me now?" I said,
            "I don't know, you know what happens when you take a lot
            of pills you shouldn't take." He asked, "Is there any-
            thing you can do?" I said, "If you ask me, I could save
            your life. But if you don't want me to, I am not going to
            bother." He thought for a while, said, "Would you save my
            life?" Then I took a bottle of Ipecac, poured the whole
            little bottle into him, and it all came out. I related
            the story to Dr. R. (the Neurologist who is following
            Milton) the next day and he said that it was the only thing
            I could have done. I acted very calm as if it didn't bother

me a bit--although I was dying inside. The next day he had completely forgotten it!

Mr. S.   We can have a violent argument, and a little while later we are buddy buddy, buddy. He just will not remember anything of what happened even though I am still steaming inside.

Dr. C.   How has this affected your own plans?

Mr. S.   This has restricted us, too, in advancing ourselves.

Mrs. S.   Yes, I would have been an Assistant Principal by now.

Mr. S.   She would have been an Assistant Principal. Maybe I would have had a bigger business, but we have been so involved with the situations that we've had and have, that we can't advance ourselves that much.

Mrs. S.   You know, two years ago I finally finished my master's degree. I started, and I had to stop. I started, and I had to stop.

Mr. S.   She still doesn't have a driver's license. She has attempted that a few times, and always gave it up in disgust because Milton would get sick, or something like what happened a few years ago. He would get so sick and end up in the hospital, and she would say "To hell with the driver's licence" you know, "to hell with that." Also in my business, "To hell with it," you know. Maybe buying some property, or a store, or something like that. You just can't maneuver as much when you have sick children.
            That's what I wanted to get across. That really restricts you.

Mrs. S.   It restricts the whole family, and it restricts each person. I found also that relatives don't invite you over when you have a case like Milton.

Mr. S.   No they don't want you in their house.

Dr. C.   So it restricts you also in terms of your social life.

Mrs. S.   Oh certainly!

Mr. S.   I remember years ago, my father had a stroke and it was very bad. His brother came over and saw him, and was really shaken up by it. His wife later on said, "I don't want my husband to see him--makes him very ill." And, of course, the same thing applies to Milton when he goes

over to somebody's house and gets an asthma attack and I
have to give him a shot. It sort of scares these people,
and they wouldn't invite us over anymore.

Dr. C.   So there are profound ways in which this has and continues
          to affect you....

Mrs. S.   They don't invite you to any weddings, bar mitzvahs, what-
          ever. We don't go anymore. If Milton can't come, we don't
          go. If he is not invited, we do not go.

Dr. C.   Has that stopped invitations?

Mr. S.   Oh yes! It has! But I don't care. One cousin had a wed-
          ding last year. I met him about two years before, and he
          said, "Wherever you go, Milton can come"; but when his
          daughter got married and he made a big wedding of 300 peo-
          ple, there wasn't room for Milton. And if there wasn't
          room for Milton, we wouldn't go. So we refused to go.
          But then after that he said he was sorry that he didn't
          ask Milton to come. He apologized.

Dr. C.   I was just going to ask you whether it hurts, but it
          sounds more like it has made you angry.

Mrs. S.   It makes you angry, but it hurts, too. It hurts, but I
          don't care. I have my standard too.

Mr. S.   It hurts him, my cousin, more.

Mrs. S.   There is nothing more important to us than Milton. He
          goes to a wedding, or to an affair, he has a great time,
          and he is good.

Dr. C.   (turning to the husband) How about enlarging your
          business?

Mr. S.   I think it restricted it.

Dr. C.   I mean now--what is stopping you now?

Mr. S.   Well, no I am tired of thinking. I can't think about it.
          It is too late. I do have other plans of being in Cali-
          fornia. We may go out there some day to settle. Even for
          Milton the climate out there might be better. Not the
          cold weather. I hope my wife is finishing up her time at
          teaching....

Mrs. S.   Not yet. I would go nuts staying home.

Mr. S.   No, not to stay home, I mean in the City, she could finish
            up her 25 years.

Mrs. S.   Then I would have to go into business. We run a flea mar-
            ket too, you know.

Mr. S.   We are busy seven days a week.

Mrs. S.   We do it every Sunday and sometimes on Saturdays.

Dr. C.   Milton goes with you sometimes?

Mr. S.   Oh, yes he comes with us. It's a good outlet for him.
            Sunday mornings we are out of the house at 7:30 in the
            morning till 6 o'clock at nights. And we are dog tired
            all the time. It's a healthy outlet for him. It's very
            good.

Dr. C.   And is it financially remunerative?

Mr. S.   Oh yes. It's very productive. Sometimes very productive.
            We do well--sweaters, and aprons and things like that.

Dr. C.   Is it a continuation of the business that you now have?

Mr. S.   Well, this is separate, entirely separate.

Mrs. S.   The business is with his brother. They are partners.
            This is our own. The other children can always use a few
            extra dollars. In fact, Melvin complains, "Don't buy me
            anymore clothes." But things are very expensive. They
            can always use the extra money. We like to help them out,
            you, you know, graduate school, a new family, they can
            always....

Mr. S.   Milton enjoys it. Before we had the flea market, we would
            be home Sunday. We would go out for rides. We would go
            to Jersey. We would go all over, but after a while, you
            could get tired of doing that. You can't stay home with
            Milton. You just can't. You can't stay home with Milton
            and sit and watch T.V. or do anything. He is constantly in
            your hair. He'll start an argument with you all the time.

Mrs. S.   Oh boy can he argue!

Dr. C.   And the flea market situation...

Mr. S.   He goes off by himself.

<u>Mrs. S.</u>   Sometimes he stays and helps, but most of the time he likes
              to just walk around, see what's there, look at this, look
              at that. He enjoys it. He just loves being out in the
              air. On the coldest day, he just loves it.

<u>Dr. C.</u>   It sounds fantastic. It sounds like you are really finding
              a productive way of coping!

Several themes now clearly emerge--themes that bespeak of unresolved and perhaps unresolvable conflicts, and to use Erickson's
designations, of stagnation instead of generativity, of despair rather than ego integrity. The deadly anger and rage at Milton and at
the interminable nature of his chronic illness are a stark contrast
to their willingness to "bargain" and keep their first son, even if
blind, if only he didn't die. Painful to see is their stagnation
and despair--not getting a driver's license, not expanding the
store, not getting a vice principalship, losing closeness with the
extended family. Until recently, they had stagnated as a response
to the stress of Milton's illness. Some movement--mother getting
her master's degree, the family project of the flea market, speaks
to some developing flexibility and a beginning renewal of their more
productive lives.

Summary and Conclusion

The S. family has shared two devastatingly painful experiences
with us--the first, the death of their oldest son from cancer, the
second, the incapacitating chronic but nonterminal illness of their
youngest son. The parents feel grey-embittered, depressed, using
Erikson's formulation, stagnant and despairing, quite in contrast
to their response to the first experience. Both events clearly altered the life course of the family--after the first, they were
able to attend to the task of generativity--the second has had a
more ominous and devastating effect on the family. This deviation
of their life course is, I feel, of pathological proportions.

The challenge of medical illness to the development of family
theory points out that we must go beyond family therapy techniques,
somehow beyond the paradigm of psychopathology to encompass the vast
array of responses of the emotionally "healthy," the emotionally
"vulnerable," and the emotionally "disturbed" to the slings and ar-
rows of outrageous nature. In this family, one parameter, that of
development even in the first approximation made by Erikson, is
used as a way of starting to think about the long term effects of
some of the medical illnesses we are considering.

Ultimately, we need to predict which families need interventions, yet not only for some time limited experiences like grief.
Before we can intelligently address this, however, we need data,
data that can be gathered under some sort of family theory that will

help us make some of these essential determinations. I feel we need
to embark on what can be called grandchild legacy research--long
term follow up of families to begin to plot a lifelong pattern following catastrophic events. In this family, we have a 23 year follow-
up and a 10 year follow-up on the death of the first and the incapacitation of their fourth child.

In deference to the superb work that Drs. Flomenhaft, Kaplan
and Langsley (1969) did about outpatient services as alternatives to
hospitalization in their Denver study, I promised Dr. Flomenhaft I
would not invoke the ghost of Dorthea Dix. However, this case does
raise important questions. If, as a society, we had decided to emphasize the development of good chronic mental hospitals and residences, perhaps on a par with those described in the middle of the
19th century during the height of the moral period of psychiatry,
adding some of the knowledge and techniques we have acquired in the
past century, it is quite likely that that outcome would have been
pursued for Milton. Deleted from the tape of the parents for this
presentation is a brief reference by the parents to the asthma
center's recommendation at the end of the first hosptalization that
institutionalization of Milton should be considered. A similar recommendation was not made two years later by the same group during
the height of the deinstitutionalization euphoria.

Had we been able to predict the outcome for this family with
Milton living at home for these ten years, an outcome that we must
eventually be able to predict if we ever develop a science of family
development, I feel some of us would have recommended some form of
residence or institution for Milton. In our emphasis on family
therapy, on crisis intervention, and on deinstitutionalization, the
long term cost to the family is easily overlooked. Perhaps it is
time for even that pendulum to begin to swing back?

REFERENCES

Berlin, I. Family Treatment of Chronic Illness in a Child. Mutual
     Developmental Problems. This Volume, Section 1.
Christ, G. Dys-synchrony of Coping Among Children, Family, and
     Staff in a Cancer Hospital. This Volume, Section 4
Erikson, E. H. Eight Ages of Man. In: Childhood and Society, W. W.
     Norton & Company, New York, 1963.
Flomenhaft, K., Kaplan, D. M. & Langsley, D. G. Avoiding Psychiatric
     Hospitalization. Social Work, 14:4, October 1969, pp. 38-45.

GHOSTS IN THE FAMILY: DISCUSSION OF DR. CHRIST'S PAPER

Peter Dunn, M.D.

Director of Family Therapy, Department of Psychiatry

Downstate Medical Center - KCHC, Brooklyn, NY

There is something about being in a family session that can lead you to forget about the ghosts in the room, family members who have died but are still very much part of the family's life drama. I want to thank Dr. Christ for this opportunity to comment upon his very moving presentation, which places in the foreground a family ghost, a 27 month old boy who died in 1956, and highlights his impact upon the family in 1980. In conceptualizing this case Dr. Christ invokes Erikson's paradigm of developmentally successive levels of system organization, each inextricably linked to earlier adaptations. His tape convincingly underlines his point. We see how flaw lines in the family's reintegration around the crisis of the death of their first child, do not emerge until nine years later in the transactions around the youngest son's asthma and later his brain damage.

Dr. Christ is correct, I believe, in using the case example to point to family therapy's difficulty in finding a place for the past in its theoretical underpinnings. Ghosts have never done well in family therapy. It may be that family therapists felt that they were being sufficiently well cared for by psychoanalysts or that the very atmosphere of a family session, with its high concentration of talk and movement, was not thought to be hospitable enough to allow them to breathe and come alive again. This is not to say that ghosts have been totally ignored. Norman Paul's (1967) emphasis on unresolved mourning and Nagy's (1973) on transgenerational legacies have always received a willing ear, but it was hard to integrate their contributions into the mainstream of family systems theory. As Dr. Christ points out these efforts have more often been regarded as technical contributions (e.g. operational mourning) than as building blocks of a more sophisticated view of the way in which families transform as they progress through the life cycle and through the generations.

Indeed it is only in the past several years that family thera-pists have come to regard the normal family as a system in continu-ing evolution. The family life cycle's developmental perspective has come to replace the prior emphasis on the family as a structured system more or less frozen in the face of the changes of time (i.e. homeostatic). Dr. Christ correctly points out the need to enrich the family developmental model by addressing the ways in which dif-ficulties (as well as opportunities) at one stage in the family life cycle draw from events and family responses of previous stages and previous generations.

No event illustrates more vividly the impact of a family's history on its subsequent unfolding than the death of a child. Such an inheritance overwhelms the human ability to mourn and must in-evitably influence all future transactions among the surviving family members until it is "washed out" over the course of several genera-tions. The surviving children become the focus of adaptive maneuvers made by the family in the creation of a new family balance. In the present case, one wonders if the parents' fears, anger, resentments and guilt about their dead child did not lead to a reflexive over-reaction to their youngest son's asthmatic wheezing. At some point a positive feedback loop was set in effect. The parents' anxiety came to exacerbate the very symptoms that they were fearful of eliciting. The whole scenario may have represented for the family the endless reenactment of the trauma of the death of the first child. Dr. Christ is quite convincing in maintaining that it is not possible to understand his patients history and present situation without reference to the dead sibling - though this is not to imply that the transactions around the boy's asthma and brain damage have not also subserved more contemporary family functions, such as the subtle monitoring of the parents' relationship.

Of course, this is not the only type of miscarried adaptation observed by those who have counseled families who have lost a child. In other families a veil of silence comes to fall on all references to the dead child, distancing family members in the service of con-taining grief. In still other families a sibling is chosen as a replacement. Such replacement children - they have been termed, "the living dead" - repetitively experience a blurring of their identities as their families attempt to reembody the dead child in their being. Again, all such maneuverings must be understood both horizontally, in terms of the family's needs in the here and now, as well as vertically, as a manifestations of the family's fixation at a point of trauma at a previous point of the life cycle. And we must be aware as in Dr. Christ's case that the pathogenic impact of the particular adaptation may not be felt for many years afterwards when the family is grappling with developmental issues seemingly far removed from the initial loss.

Health care practioners called upon to counsel families who have endured the death of child would be mindful to study this case. In a field replete with anectodal reports of initial interviews and other "brief encounters" we must be grateful to Dr. Christ for allowing us this twenty-three year panoramic view of the shadow cast by a child's death and illness on the subsequent life of his family.

BIBLIOGRAPHY

Paul, N. The role of mourning and empathy in conjoint family therapy. In Family Therapy and Disturbed Families, G. Zuk & I. Boszormenyi-Nagy (Eds.), Science and Behavior Books, Palo Alto, CA, 1967, pp. 186-206.

Boszormenyi-Nagy & Spark, G.M. Invisible Loyalties: Reciprocity in Intergenerational Family Therapy, Harper & Row, New York, NY, 1973.

MOURNING AND PARENTECTOMY: GENERAL DISCUSSION

Dr. Henry Schneer: Audience Member, Child Psychiatrist

I was fascinated with how Dr. Christ enabled Melvin to mobilize his aggression. Henry Peskin, (the well known specialist on
asthma), used to advise that there be a parentectomy which consisted of sending the child away from the parent to an asthma center as was done in this case. My question is: What experience has
there been with the use of family therapy as an alternative to that
kind of drastic parentectomy?

Dr. Christ

I am not aware of any research that completely answers your
question, Dr. Schneer. One part can be answered: The group mentioned in this case found great improvement in all children with
asthma whom they hospitalized, except the steroid dependent asthmatic youngsters. Minuchin and his co-workers, using structured
family therapy, were able to reduce the severity of the asthma;
indeed they were able to reduce or eliminate the steroids, in a significant number of steroid-dependent asthmatic children. Here is a
group where parentectomy did not, but family therapy did, improve by
an alteration of the family interaction.

Dr. Sargent

There is about an 85% improvement in the kids with reduction
or elimination of steroid use through the use of structural family
therapy over a six to nine month time period.

Audience Member

My feeling as I watch the tape was that perhaps the time for a
parentectomy is now? Is that part of the work that's still to be
done?

Audience Member

In the case that Dr. Christ presented, I would like to focus

on a different perspective: I felt very overwhelmed by the events
in the family's life. Even if we eliminate the death of the first
child, and look only at Melvin, the youngest son, he presents an
overwhelming task even to a family which, like this one, has no major
psychopathology. The amount of energy that is continuously expanded
by the parents in setting limits, by confronting issues like his
suicidal threats, must be overwhelming. The parents must find this
an intolerable existential situation. In the past, we accepted institutionalization much more readily. I feel that our emphasis on
a community oriented family oriented approach does major injustice
to families like the S's.

Dr. Christ

Although your question goes counter to the zeitgeist of current popular psychiatric thinking, it is nevertheless an extremely
important question. Although the parents have the emotional strength
to recognize, even acknowledge on the videotape, that they have at
times wished for the boy's death, and on the recommendation of the
Pediatrician sent the boy to the asthma center for two years, they
are not at all prepared to place permanently their son.

I am afraid that the strong anti-hospitalization ethnic has not
fostered a full scale development of a variety of permanent residences. The cost to the family of keeping the boy at home has been
very great. They now are starting to mobilize their emotional and
cognitive resources to get on with the business of adult development - but their plans clearly include taking care of the boy. Were
there good affordable residences or state hospitals that could
promise optimal care and optimize further development of their son,
they might gradually reconsider. However, they haven't crossed that
bridge yet. I'm certain that they would not allow their other two
children to assume the burden of caring for Melvin. As they enter
old age, and foresee their own life end, I'm certain they will seek
other solutions for the boy.

Dr. John Tsiouris: Audience Member, Child Psychiatrist

My question is addressed to Dr. Dunn. In reference to the
family presented by Dr. Christ, there were really two ghosts in this
family. One was the ghost of the dead child and the other one was
the ghost of the still living but now very altered child. Is there
any difference in the impact of these two different ghosts on the
family?

Dr. Dunn

There are two mournings that haven't been completed in the family. One is for Melvin's lost personality because he underwent a
total personality reorganization, and the other mourning was for the

child who died but who hadn't been mourned. The loss of a body
part requires the kind of mourning that in many ways is similar to
the loss of a person. There are very similar dynamics that go on
but different techniques for working with it. You can mourn a real
person who died with the whole family in a way that facilitates the
affect coming out and is progressive which cannot be done with a
child like Melvin who has undergone a personality change. This is
an issue to be addressed with the whole family.

Dr. Christ

    I can only agree with part of Dr. Dunn's interpretation. In-
deed, the parents cannot mourn the loss of Melvin's personality and
potential. In part, it is as if there are two Melvins - the 7 year
old bright boy they sent to the asthma center for help with his
asthma and the retarded young man who is now living with them and
who is so extraordinarily difficult to manage. The parents cannot
accept that the bright, eager, curious personable Melvin is dead as
they "keep looking for a miracle".

    As to the first child, I feel they have mourned him. I'm not
sure parents can ever fully bury and forget their child. The son
will remain alive in their memory as long as they live especially,
as they say, during certain anniversaries, even at unexpected moments when the memories are vividly recalled as was done by me in
the interview. Their emotions were deeply felt, but the mourning
of parents for their child will always retain deep, undistorted,
undefended feelings of longing, of sadness for the lost potential,
of sadness at the death of their hopes and aspirations.

"DIS-SYNCHRONY" OF COPING AMONG CHILDREN WITH CANCER, THEIR FAMILIES,

AND THE TREATING STAFF

Grace Christ, M.S.W.

Memorial Sloan-Kettering Cancer Center

New York, New York

"Dis-synchrony" in coping refers to an occurrence at different points in time of unevenness in specific cognitive appraisals or affective states of parent and patient, parent and parent, patient and sibling, and patient, family, and staff. In this presentation, I will discuss the role of the mental health worker in facilitating or enabling communication and synchrony, or in Dr. Kaplan's terms, "mediating the stresses" caused by a lack of synchrony (Kaplan, 1973). Several vignettes will be presented which demonstrate some interventions between a mother and her nine year old daughter.

Cancer in children used to be an acute illness which lasted months instead of years, and was followed by the child's death. In most cases, this is no longer the situation. With the advent of the use of multiple chemotherapeutic agents, new surgical techniques and new uses of radiation, children with leukemia have achieved a five year survival rate of about 50%, with osteogenic sarcoma 50%, and with Hodgkins disease 85%. However, the treatment protocols confront both patient and family with enormous physical and emotional stresses over long periods of time. At the end of the siege, the child may die, or live to face the problems of reorienting goals and of continuing to live with the constant threat of recurrence.

At this point in time, it is more precise to think of child-hood cancer as a chronically acute illness, affecting the patient and family over many years, and requiring complex and diverse coping strategies at various points in the process. Throughout this process there may be vast differences in family members' understanding of what is happening, and why it is happening, as well as differences in the timing of emotional responses. This lack of synchrony in

85

cognitive appraisal and in emotional responses can cause enormous distress among family members, and should be a priority focus for mental health workers seeking to enhance family adaptation to what is usually a dreadful sequence of events.

At Memorial Sloan-Kettering Cancer Center, 57% of the 1500 pediatric patients are from the New York City Metropolitan area and New York State, 23% from New Jersey, 10% from out the United States. This means families are often split, members are separated from their support networks, that is, people who would ordinarily be intimately involved in serious illness or family problems and who would be able to enhance clarification of information and perception, emotional reaction, and provide emotional support. This places an added burden on the treatment team in a medical center even with intact families who demonstrate good coping abilities and resilience.

While the probability of discrepant views and lack of synchrony is greater in patients and families with prior psychopathology, it may occur in any family, brought on by the stresses of the situation. I am using this particular word "dis-synchrony" because it avoids the implication of psychopathology that so many other terms and concepts such as skewed, enmeshed, schismatic, pseudo-mutual, etc. evoke (Guerin, 1976). And yet, it still allows us to address problems in adaptation that require intervention by the mental health worker. The predominantly psychiatrically oriented mental health professional's tendency to focus on psychopathology is perhaps one of the most striking examples of dis-synchrony between oncologist, medically ill patients and their families. Behavior and symptoms are automatically viewed in terms of the psychopathology they may represent in the psychiatrically disturbed, rather than seen in the perspective of their function in the process of adaptation to the crisis of illness in an otherwise emotionally healthy individual. Regression, denial, even illusion, may be powerful coping defenses at certain points in the treatment process. Acute stress, however, can result when the specific coping efforts of one family member are out of synchrony with another. I will describe later in this paper the dis-synchrony brought about by one mother's need to control her own reaction to her daughter's serious illness by denying access of information to her child in order to control her own confrontation by the facts. It became clear that the mother's hysterical characterological style served to prevent her own emotional overwhelm. The dis-synchrony is evident when we keep in mind that, in contrast to the mother's need to minimize information, the patient needed to learn all the details of her illness and treatment, making adaptive use of the latency defense of intellectualization.

Our experience is that family service agencies and psychiatric clinics generally either refuse to see our families on an ongoing

basis, or they begin treatment but refuse to find out about or integrate knowledge of the realistic impact of the illness on the
patient and on the family's current functioning. They take the
stance that the patient's emotional reactions are no different from
those of any other emotionally disturbed patient they treat. This
unwillingness to reorient one's appraisal and perspective to include
the essential dimension of the medical illness is not limited to
cancer. I recently observed an initial family interview with a
16 year old boy with hemophilia, his 12 year old sister, 14 year
old brother, mother and formerly alcoholic father. This interview
was conducted in a nationally prominent family agency by two co-
therapists, one of them a psychiatrist. Mental health workers
regardless of their discipline tend to underestimate the importance
of a sophisticated knowledge of the medical disease. The patient
had begun failing school subsequent to a medical crisis in which he
had almost died. The family members and the patient demonstrated
confusion regarding facts about the illness, the genetic cause of
the illness, including who were carriers of the disease, as well
as facts about the recent medical crisis. The mother, but not
the 16 year old patient, was communicating with the hematologist,
which was contributing to the patient's lack of knowledge. The
school was unclear about how far they should push the patient to
attend and perform. In the discussion, after the family session,
the therapists demonstrated their own confusion about many aspects
of the illness and its treatment. However, they were resistant
to exploring these medical facts. Instead, they focused on the
interpersonal dynamics, alliances, structures etc. At the same time,
they stated they were eager to work with these kinds of families
because they were engaging and often made rapid progress.

It has been our experience that, indeed, families whose problems
are primarily related to dis-synchrony of coping can accommodate
rather quickly to clarification of differing needs, perceptions, and
coping styles. However, inadequate factual information about the
disease, its course, and the reality stresses it produces, seriously
reduces the effectiveness of the interventions, and indeed can
iatrogenically, produce stress.

Ten years of my own professional work was with families who
sought mental health interventions for problems of severe psychopathology, seven with families of adolescents, hospitalized for
mental illness with Jim Masterson, M.D. at Payne Whitney (Masterson,
1972), and three with autistic and schizophrenic younger children
with their parents in Mahler's Masters' Research Center (Mahler,
1968). These families were clearly much more fixed in their coping
patterns than the vast majority of the families who are being treated
on our Pediatrics Service. Our families are distressed and demonstrate disturbed and disturbing behavior patterns, on the surface
often indistinguishable from symptoms seen in chronically disturbed

families. However, they often seek out help, and respond quickly
to a variety of individual and group interventions, and do not require the type and extent of psychotherapy as do the emotionally
disturbed families.

While it is true that cancer is a leveler, and that the proportion of severely emotionally disturbed, vulnerable, and normal
reflects the incidence of such states in the total population, we
need to look at the continuum of coping behaviors in people rather
than only in the emotionally disturbed extremes. Our task as mental
health professionals is to understand the crises of illness, its
impact on patient and family, the variety of modes of adaptation,
and how we can be of help not only with those therapeutic tools
useful to the emotionally disturbed, but to modify our approaches
commensurate with the needs and strengths of the severely trauma-
tized nonemotionally disturbed population.

PARENT-YOUNG CANCER PATIENT DIS-SYNCHRONY

One of the most common "dis-synchronies" is that between the
parent and the young child. Parents often cling to the belief that
the young child is oblivious to the seriousness of the illness. So,
for example, at Memorial, we have a play therapy group for children,
giving them the opportunity to use medical equipment and rubber
puppets to abreact, clarify, raise questions and get information
about the medical procedures they are undergoing. The social worker
talks with the parents ahead of time to find out what they have
told the child about the illness and what they think the patient
understands. Often, the parents will say the child knows very
little, and certainly nothing about the seriousness of the illness.
However, the worker usually finds, through observing the child's
play, that, indeed, he knows many details about the illness and its
treatment.

The play group is a good way to assess children's fantasies and
misperceptions about what is happening to them. The worker asked a
five year old patient why he had an I.V. in his arm. He explained
that the I.V. kept him pumped up so that he looked like a normal
boy. If they took the I.V. out, he would go down like a balloon.
Another patient revealed his thought that he was in the hospital
because his mother had just come home with a new baby which she
liked better, so she had traded him in. A third patient said he
thought this happened to him because he was delayed in toilet
training: "I peed too much." Such fantastic misconstructions should
be watched for particularly in the child at the preoperational stage
of development during which "magical" "animistic" thinking is
expected, i.e., age two - seven. Additionally, Piaget described the
child's inability to realize on his own the presence of such dis-
tortion (Christ, 1977). Hence, one must not expect the child to

request clarification. He will accept such fantastic explanations as factual.

Some information, on the other hand, is often amazingly accurate. During one play group, one of the patients "called a code" on a doll. The other patients rushed to help. One patient started an I.V., another a respirator, and a third began pounding on the doll's chest. They called for blood and instruments. Suddenly, the lead child stopped and announced, "It's o.k.; he's going to make it," much to the therapist's relief. "Calling a code" is one of the more dramatic events in a hospital when heroic measures such as those used by the children are required to revive an otherwise acutely dying patient on the floor.

It is interesting to observe that adults are often disturbed by the degree of aggression displayed in the play group. Some of the doctors still become upset when they see the doctor and nurse puppets so badly abused. "Don't you reassure them," they ask, "that we are really trying to help?" This is, of course, done repeatedly, but that does not alter the fact that the normal aggression and hostility of children in this situation is very real and needs expression and acceptance.

One intervention we have used to help parents become more aware of their child's understanding of the illness is to video tape the child's play sessions with the puppets and medical equipment. The parents then observe the tape. Nine year old Joanna had been diagnosed with leukemia two months prior to the taping. Mrs. B., her mother, had insisted throughout this period that Joanna did not know the name of her illness, and very reluctantly agreed to Joanna's participation in the routine teaching of children about their illness by the nursing staff on the service. Staff was concerned about Joanna because she was quite depressed and there seemed to be an uncomfortable distance between her and her mother. Although Mrs. B. was conscientious about the physical care of the child, she seemed emotionally aloof from Joanna, as well as being distant from her own feelings of grief and loss. Joanna demonstrated in her play an intimate and detailed knowledge of her illness, treatment, and the many procedures she had to undergo. Her anger about what was being done to her body was demonstrated in continuous stories of sick doctors and nurses who had "blood problems" and who required numerous painful procedures which Joanna eagerly administered. At one point in the play, she described a child getting hurt because she disobeyed her parents. The social worker explained that many children think they are sick because of something bad they have done. Sadly Joanna said she too thought she was sick because of things she had done wrong to her mother or family, but her mother had explained that was not true. "Some children have to get sick...no they don't have to, they just do."

Following observation of the tape, Mrs. B. spoke more openly about her anger at what had happened to Joanna, and of her rage at the children who teased her in school one day about her bald head. While she was impressed with the knowledge Joanna had gained about her illness, she wishes that Joanna "didn't know any of it," that her mind could be occupied with more normal information for a child her age. She reported feeling better following the observation of the tape, stating she "got in touch with" feelings she had been hiding and, indeed, seemed more relaxed and comfortable around Joanna.

Although the mother has had numerous stresses in her life, two seriously ill children, and an alcoholic husband, she has in fact coped very well. Initially reluctant to allow Joanna to be taught about her illness, she agreed after only one session with the nurses and one with myself during which she worked through her fears and apprehensions.

I had seven more formal interviews in the course of the next twelve months with Mrs. B. before she moved with her parents to California to be close to her brother, a successful lawyer. During that time, her father had been diagnosed with colon cancer, and her divorce was finalized. Mrs. B. used our sessions to talk over problems presented by illness, consequent changes in her life style, and past conflicts reawakened and brought into new perspective by the current crisis. I am bringing this out to document how a normal parent can use brief, but as Dr. Kaplan points out, timely intervention to enable them to survive through crises. Mrs. B. reached out to me when Joanna had a toxic reaction to chemotherapy, when her divorce was finalized, when her father was diagnosed with cancer, when she experienced problems in dating, and when she was preparing to tell her doctor she was moving to California. Some authors talk about being available to the normally coping parent. I think what is needed is something more than passive availability, but much less than ongoing intensive psychotherapy. There needs to be an ongoing interaction with parents focused by the worker's monitoring of the family's coping processes around those predictably stressful times in the course of illness and in those normally stressful life events that are complicated by the illness.

PARENT-ADOLESCENT PATIENT DIS-SYNCHRONY

With the adolescent patient, the dis-synchrony often has to do with the increased dependence of the patient on the parent just at the point where each parent and adolescent is beginning to feel somewhat free from the struggles of the second individuation-separation stage of development. The parent struggles with anger at the adolescent's regression and the loss of the normal child, and the adolescent struggles with the terror of the illness, which often enhances dependency at the very point when his need for stage-specific independence is in ascendence. What is often required by the mental health worker is an initial acceptance of this regression to a more dependent, less assertive independence, and a more gradual enhancement of the separate identity and movement toward individuation by encouraging mastery and self-awareness, usually through greater knowledge about the illness, i.e., the use of intellectualization as a stage specific defense.

Fifteen year old Marcy had bone replacement surgery for osteogenic sarcoma. The staff was alarmed by the degree of control Marcy's mother exerted over her, and the hostility the mother expressed to which Marcy seemed unable to respond. Staff wanted Marcy to speak up for herself, or at least to be critical of her mother. "Don't they understand," she confided in me, "she's all I've got." Marcy had not completed the normal process of separation. Illness was perceived as punishment for independent strivings, and the loss of mother was felt to be the loss of self and of existence, i.e., dying. This example represents a dys-synchrony in views between patient, family, and staff, and perhaps a lack of empathy on the staff's part for what it was like to be in the patient's bed.

An example of touching empathy and synchrony was demonstrated by the mother of a 12 year old who was in the last days of the terminal phase of osteogenic sarcoma. Although the patient was semi-comatose, she was having memories of traumatic events in her early childhood which indeed had been violent. Her father was murdered a year before she was diagnosed with cancer and had abused her mother when the patient was a young child. As the patient reviewed these events in her early life, the mother was able to listen, remember, clarify facts, and reassure her daughter of her continuing presence and of her protection as she was dying. The social worker in this case made herself available to the mother for abreaction, clarification and reality testing, following these extremely difficult, yet most important sessions of mutual review of the girl's early life experiences.

DIS-SYNCHRONY BETWEEN PATIENT AND SIBLINGS AND PARENT AND SIBLINGS

The fathers were the neglected group in the child guidance clinics. The siblings often seem to have that position in the acute care hospital. As cancer patients are living longer with stressful treatment, the suffering of the siblings may be even greater than when patients died more quickly. Their reactions and the level at which they can be engaged, will have a lot to do with their own developmental level and their previous and current relationship to the patient. Parents are often oblivious to the concerns and problems of the siblings. Suddenly a problem will surface--usually a school difficulty--that has clearly been going on for some time. Parents are so preoccupied with the physical,

mental, and emotional demands of the cancer patient that they
cannot allow the possibility of difficulty which would potentially
ask more of them. The parents' exhaustion is real. But the needs
of the siblings are also very real.

The parents' unavailability to the sibling and unawareness
of what is really heppening to them is the rule rather than the
exception. Therefore, the mental health professional must actively
encourage and help parents keep in touch with their other children.
There is an amazing lack of information about the effects of long
term chronic illness on the siblings. What studies have been done
have focused on the siblings' reactions to death rather than the
effects of the illness and treatment. Factors identified that seem
to affect how siblings react to death include the age of the sibling,
the prevailing relationship, the course of the illness itself, the
amount of communication about the illness in the family early in
the course of treatment.

There is also very little in the literature about the changes
in the relationship between patients and siblings (Saurkes, 1980).
Some extraordinary demonstrations of synchrony and empathy as well
as the painful affects of dis-synchrony are shown in the following
examples. Parents of six year old Cheryl told the social worker
of their concern about her refusal to go to school while eight year
old Bert was in the hospital. Cheryl believed Bert was already
dead and could not be reassured by her parents. Indeed, Bert was
not doing well. The worker encouraged them to bring her in to visit
Bert. "I know this is the last time I'll be seeing you," she
announced to Bert, "because I know you are dying. I want you to
know that I love you." "I love you too," Bert replied, "and I
want you to know you can have my Legos." Cheryl returned to school
following her visit to her brother.

The three friends of an adolescent boy demonstrated unusual
empathy. They appeared in the clinic one day with the patient who
had become bald from the chemotherapy, all three with their own
heads shaved.

The next example highlights one of the most difficult areas
of dis-synchrony for adolescent patients and their siblings. The
patients struggle desperately to hold on to areas of similarity and
sameness with siblings, while siblings, out of fear, often distance
themselves and emphasize differences. One patient, who was a
twin, had lost a leg from amputation and his hair from chemotherapy.
He said to his social worker who was going to the lobby to meet
his brother, "You'll recognize him because he looks just like me."

Loss of communication with a sibling can be very painful to
patients. One 13 year old girl with osteogenic sarcoma said sadly
of her 15 year old brother, "We used to talk about everything, now

he is quiet and when I talk about being sick, he changes the subject." A 17 year old male patient with an amputation stated of his
16 year old brother, "We used to be very competitive in sports--we
fought a lot. Now I can't compete without my leg, and I'm in the
hospital so much of the time. He can't really understand my treatment, and I don't know about the things he is doing now. I wish we
could fight again."

Siblings' withdrawal from the patient may result in misconceptions about the patient's illness, such as believing the disease is
contagious or that they caused it in some way, or from complicated
and mixed emotions, such as anger toward the patient for the attention he is receiving, guilt over being healthy and well, or fear of
close identification and consequent vulnerability.

This area of dis-synchrony can be addressed through early
encouragement of communication within the family about the illness,
periodic meetings with the patient and his siblings with a focus
on communication and/or the development of sibling groups.

PROBLEMS IN DIS-SYNCHRONY BETWEEN PARENT AND PARENT

The diagnosis of a child with cancer places enormous stress
on the parents individually and on the relationship between them.
Each parent must find his own way of coping with the grief, guilt
and rage, and come to some agreement with the spouse about the
division of labor in relation to the many new physical as well as
emotional tasks confronting them. Additional time spent by one
spouse with the sick child in hospital over many months pulls the
couple apart physically, psychologically and emotionally. These
differences in tasks performed and in ways of coping can cause
enormous stress on both parents and patient and can contribute to
parental emotional exhaustion or emotional overwhelm. This is often
most clearly seen at the point of terminal illness. As the child
ceases to respond to conventional treatments, decisions have to be
made by the parents with the medical staff about how long to continue
trying research drugs. If the mother has been in the hospital with
the child, accumulating medical information, and seeing the effects
of new drugs on other patients, she may be ready to discontinue
active treatment before the father, who has been away from hospital,
working one, sometimes two jobs. The father often wants to keep
trying because he is not yet ready to accept the child's death. The
father's sense of helplessness and inadequacy at this point may be
increased by the fact that his knowledge of the medical situation is
now much less than his wife's. The staff may also unwittingly
exclude the father, because it takes so much longer to explain
things to him than to his more medically sophisticated wife. Finally,
at times the mother herself excludes the father as an expression of
her anger at having to be so predominantly responsible for the
child's treatment in the hospital and her desperate need to feel some

sense of control.

The social worker needs to clarify these areas of dis-synchrony
so she can then help the parents to join in the final decision making
tasks. She also needs to encourage staff to make a special effort
to include the father in any discussion, directing questions and
comments to him.

At the terminal stage of the illness, either or both parents may
prematurely or excessively withdraw from the patient. This can be
viewed as an expression of parental ambivalence and abandonment or
as a consequence of emotional exhaustion or emotional overwhelm.
The latter is much more often the case. It is all too easy for the
staff to blame the parents in any pediatric situation. As the child
is dying, the pressure to find someone to blame for this dreadful
turn of events is extraordinary. Psychiatric labeling of parents
can be the staff's way of casting blame and coping with their own
helplessness and despair. This must be strongly guarded against.
If the parent is exhausted or overwhelmed, it is the role and
responsibility of the mental health worker to find new supplies and
provide supportive interventions that enable parents, patient, and
staff to complete their tasks with dignity. One of the most common
dis-synchronies at the point of terminal illness is one parent's need
to discuss and abreact and the other's need to emotionally distance
himself, focusing on activity. The pain of alienation and aloneness
at this point can be severe.

It is also true that in responding to the demands of the new
tasks, the parents over the sometimes lengthy course of the illness
develop new roles vis-a-vis each other. These need to be accommodated. For example, mothers from the suburbs often become expert in
negotiating the city, and in fact may begin to enjoy regular interaction with professional staff. The husband may feel uncomfortable
with and alienated by his wife's new more assertive role. These
represent areas of dis-synchrony between parents caused by the stress
of the illness and its treatment that can become salient points for
intervention by the mental health worker.

DIS-SYNCHRONY BETWEEN PATIENT/FAMILY AND STAFF

Dis-synchrony of coping between patient/family and staff can
occur throughout the course of the patient's illness, but are most
visible at the points of crisis in the illness where important
decisions have to be made. These nine crisis points include: (1)
the time of the diagnosis; (2) the beginning of treatment; (3) negative physical reactions to the treatment; (4) failure of conventional
treatment; (5) the end of a treatment protocol; (6) the recurrence or
metastasis of the disease; (7) the initiation of research treatments; (8) the termination of active treatment; and (9) the point

of terminal illness. At these times, the goals, values, and coping styles of the family can conflict with those of the treating team. One of the most frequent areas of conflict stems from the research orientation of our institution and of the treating team. The professional team has a strong desire to fight the disease as long as possible. The recurrence of the illness, that is, the failure of the treatment, is usually felt by the staff as a failure. The patients and families who come to Memorial Sloan-Kettering Cancer Center are also in favor of research goals and of fighting the disease. However, physical and emotional exhaustion may lead the patients and families to want to terminate active treatment before the physician would wish. This is a difficult decision for patients, and they are exquisitely sensitive to any sign of emotional withdrawal by the physician as a criticism or lack of acceptance of their decision.

SUMMARY

In summary, then, I have identified the phenomena of dis-synchrony of coping between children with cancer, their families, and the treating staff as an overlooked source of distress in this otherwise psychiatrically normal population. This way of describing difficulties in adaptation has the advantage of avoiding the implication of psychopathology, but enhancing the identification of problems with which the mental health worker can be helpful. A number of vignettes of these dis-synchronies have been presented. Behavior reflecting dis-synchrony can most readily be observed during the nine identified crisis points which occur in the course of the cancer patient.

The reality of staffing patterns mandates a precision and economy of intervention with patients and families in any setting. The most frequently asked question is: How do you decide to see which patients, when, and for what purpose? The dis-synchrony which occurs during the nine crisis points described in this paper is offered as a guide for parsimoniously monitoring family adaptation.

REFERENCES

Christ, A. Cognitive Assessment of the Psychotic Child: A Piagetian Perspective. Journal of the American Academy of Child Psychiatry, 16(2):227-237, 1977.

Guerin, P. Family Therapy. New York: Gardner Press, 1976.

Kaplan, D., Smith, A., and Grobstein, R. Family Mediation of Stress. Social Work, 18(4):60-69, July, 1973.

Mahler, M. S. On Human Symbiosis and the Vicissitudes of Individuation: Infantile Psychosis. Vol. 1, New York: International Universities Press, 1968.

Masterson, J. M. P. Treatment of the Borderline Adolescent: A
     Developmental Approach. New York: Wiley--Interscience, 1972.
Sourkes, B. Siblings of the Pediatric Cancer Patient. In
     J. Hellerman (Ed.) Psychological Aspects of Childhood Cancer,
     New York: Charles C. Thomas, 1980.

"THE LORD BROUGHT ME THRU"[*]: DISCUSSION OF MRS. CHRIST'S PAPER

Kushalata R. Jayakar, M.D.

Downstate Medical Center-Kings County Hospital

Brooklyn, New York

Mrs. Christ has emphasized in her presentation that cancer is a serious, life threatening, chronic illness. Even though prognosis and life expectancy have changed drastically during the last two decades, the close connection between cancer and death has not yet changed. Until this final end point is reached, treatment is often prolonged, painful, debilitating and, in certain cases, mutilating. The psychological impact of these factors has become a major focal point in the treatment of cancer by mental health professionals.

Cancer is no longer to be viewed as merely a terminal illness. Instead, it is a prolonged, stressful situation which takes a toll on both the physical and psychological resources of the patients and their families. This includes disruption of their routine life styles and imposes excessive financial hardship and, as if these were not enough, they are placed on an emotional roller coaster by periods of relapses and remissions.

Current literature addresses the effects that illness has on: parent's reactions to their children's illness; children's reactions to their own illness, hospitalizations and separations; healthy siblings' reactions to the sick or dying patient; and reactions of medical personnel who provide direct services to the child patients. Mrs. Christ points out that major problems arise because of the dis-synchrony between different people involved in this process. There is clearly a need to reduce this dis-synchrony through the intervention of mental health professionals. Dis-synchrony may come

---

[*]The author is indebted to Mr. Ira Gershansky for his valuable editorial assistance.

at different stress points during the course of the illness, and
may affect different members of the family and personnel involved
with the case differently and at different points in time. It,
therefore, becomes crucial, not only to mediate this dis-synchrony
after it comes about, but to reduce its future probability.

I would like to focus on some of the possible causative factors
of such dis-synchronies: One factor is that the illness involves
remissions and relapses which are not always of predictable duration
or intensity. As patients get accustomed to coming to the clinic
for routine blood counts and bone marrow examinations, and as these
procedures become more routine, they begin to feel relaxed. They
can begin to deny the serious outcome of their illness until suddenly
advised, for example, of a need for a lumbar puncture because CNS
Leukemia is suspected. There are some patients, on the other hand,
who feel and act as if they are awaiting a death sentence during
every visit right from the start.

Second, while dealing with these stresses, each family member
responds according to his own individual emotional characterological
style or pattern. These differ qualitatively as well as quantita-
tively, depending on how much psychic energy each person has expended
during different phases of his/her life both prior to the illness
and during the ordeal itself.

A final factor which is unique to pediatric patients is that
children are constantly changing as they grow. The child at the
onset of his illness is quite different developmentally from the
same child several weeks, months or years later, as he or she continues to be sick. Because cognitive and emotional changes during
normal growth and development have a major impact upon the way a
child is able to handle stress in general, the stress of such a grave
illness like cancer will magnify the effect of these developmental
changes. As the child develops cognitively, he becomes more aware
of the meaning of his own illness and death; and, hence, there is an
increase in the emotional pain associated with the disease. Recognition of these factors becomes the very essence of appropriate and
timely intervention.

According to a study by Merling-Peterson and McCabe (1978)
which analyzed 96 children's narratives about death, it was noted
that concerns about death were virtually absent in children between
three and one half to five years. On those occasions when there
was a mention of death, a total absence of an affective element was
noted. A clear and sudden shift was seen in the next age group
(five and one half to nine years) when concern and curiosity about
death was described. Increased exposure to death was not deemed a
sufficient explanation for such a shift. Children of this age range
begin to construct meaningful rules about their world. There is more
systematic thinking in terms of cause and effect, with a continued

absence of affective expression. Children nine years and older,
on the other hand, begin to display affect in addition to their
descriptions of death.

In clinical practice, it is noted that both children and
parents go through the emotional reactions described by Kubler-Ross
(1970), i.e., the stages of anger, denial, hope, bargaining, and
acceptance. It is therefore essential, as Mrs. Christ points out,
to anticipate the emotional reactions and make very active interventions rather than merely being passively available. When dealing
with the issues concerning the finality of death and its long lasting
effects, one cannot overemphasize the value of timely intervention
for the resolution of dynamic issues such as anger, guilt, and in
some cases, unconscious death wishes.

Finally, I would like to emphasize that as mental health
professionals, we must all come to accept the fact that death is
final and cannot be avoided. In the face of this finality, we
intellectually set up a system to take over and stay in control of
a situation over which we have no control. We look for ways and
means to make death and dying less painful and less fearful while
we continue to search for internal reserves of strength. These
strengths do exist somewhere or in someone, perhaps in the father,
mother, sister, nurses, volunteers, or in the patients themselves.
Our goal is to search for them and, once found, to utilize them to
the fullest.

I would like to end by giving a brief case vignette of a little
girl who didn't give up: Three years ago, eight year old Patty was
admitted with a severe relapse of leukemia. According to the medical
personnel, her death was imminent. Her mother at this point was
so depleted, after having gone through similar ordeals before, that
she was not even able to pray or cry. Patty kissed her mother, told
her not to worry, prayed, and said good night. The next morning
she handed me a piece of paper on which she had written the following
poem:

> Lord brought me thru, Lord brought me thru
> Yes he did.
> I can feel in my soul
> I can feel in my heart
> The Lord brought me thru--Yes he did.
> When I was blind,
> I could not see
> Jesus and Doctors rescued me
> Because I knew they would
> The Lord brought me thru--Yes he did.
> When I was sick and almost gone,
> My mother was there to make me strong

> The Lord brought me thru
> Yes he did! Yes he did!

The little girl and her mother are still visiting the clinic
regularly. She is now 11 years old. When I asked her mother's
permission to read her daughter's poem, she said with pride and
tears, "Well doctor, read it to as many people, and let them know
how my Patty never gave up, because, after all, until we die, we
got to keep on living!"

REFERENCES

Kubler-Ross, E. On Death and Dying. New York: McMillan, 1970.
Merling-Peterson, C. and McCabe, A. Children Talk about Death.
    Omega--Journal of Death and Dying, Vol. 8, 305-331, 1977.

TIMELY REACHING OUT TO FAMILIES: GENERAL DISCUSSION

Carl Bryant: Audience Member--Social Worker

I was particularly struck by Mrs. Christ's use of the concept of being more than passively available to the cancer patients and their families on an ongoing basis. I would like some discussion of specific techniques of how you do this with patients.

Mrs. Christ

It is important that the mental health professional not wait for the parent or patient to come to him with a "problem." Rather, the mental health professional should be aware of the informational and supportive needs of patients and families with different illnesses at various points in the treatment process and offer appropriate help. Further, he should know the range of coping responses in order to be able to identify extremes. For example, our social workers observe that families take about a week to ten days to work through the initial emotional shock of the diagnosis and begin to mobilize themselves to reorganize family life to meet the new demands--financially, socially, etc. This is identified as the first crisis point in my presentation. If a parent is observed to be unable to make necessary plans after two weeks, more intensive intervention is necessary, such as offering help by suggesting alternative ways of organizing their situation, suggesting where to look for resources, whom to communicate with about the illness, etc. Much important time is lost if one waits for the patient or parent to identify the problem. This does not mean, of course, that one is insensitive to varieties of coping styles. Some families are resistant to obvious efforts to help, especially with emotional reactions. However, almost all families will accept information, education and genuine statements of concern.

Nellie Sandler: Audience Member--Social Worker

Another piece of dis-synchrony that struck me is between family and hospital, particularly around utilization review. We often have families who are unable, for one reason or another, to take their

children home when the hospital needs to have the children go home.
The families' response determines whether they are then considered
as the good or the bad ones, which adds an additional piece of
stress to them.

Mrs. Christ

At Memorial Sloan-Kettering, social work is a very integral
part of the whole utilization review process. It is our experience
that it is important for the social worker to initiate contact with
the family and medical staff about planned length of stay in
hospital at the point of admission, and not wait for a referral.
Orderly transition of patients in and out of the hospital is a primary concern of the social worker. It is her job to keep the family
informed of the time frame and what is expected of them, and to
keep medical staff informed of any special problems the family may
have in caring for the patient at home and ways those may be solved.
The social worker has to be pretty active in locating resources,
home care services, financial services, etc. for families who are
experiencing some difficulty, e.g., where both parents work or
where the primary-care-taking parent is emotionally disturbed or the
home situation is disorganized or deprived.

Dr. Ake Mattsson

I want to thank Mrs. Christ and the discussant very much. As
Mrs. Christ was presenting her paper, I was struck by the potential
that the nine crisis points that she outlines can be used in a
research design. I'm sure Mrs. Christ has something like this in
mind, but I can imagine a grid where one would vertically list
coping styles, adaptive responses, successes, etc., horizontally,
family members, patients, and team members, and in a third dimension,
the nine crisis points. Could you say something about that?

Mrs. Christ

That is very perceptive! We are embarking on exactly such a
venture. The first, possibly the hardest, step is a clear definition
of each of the concepts in these three dimensions.

OPEN-HEART SURGERY FOR CONGENITAL HEART DISEASE: MINIMIZING ADVERSE

PSYCHOLOGICAL SEQUELAE IN FAMILIES FACING MAJOR HIGH-RISK SURGERY

H. Paul Gabriel, M.D. and Delores A. Danilowicz, M.D.

New York University School of Medicine

New York, New York

Ever since the original studies of Spitz (1945), Bowlby (1960), Robertson (1958), and Anna Freud, there has been a growing awareness that separation, hospitalization, and illness of any kind represent a major crisis in the life of a child. However, only in recent years has the immense importance of the family been recognized as essential to the child's care and prevention of serious psychological sequelae after illness. In addition, the advances of modern medicine and the complexity of the tertiary care hospital have turned certain types of major illnesses into a unique and unusual set of experiences for children and families. Certainly this is true of those illnesses that at one time were uniformly or predominantly fatal in early childhood.

Before the introduction of new techniques and as a result of studies in institutions and hospitals (Spitz, 1945; Robertson, 1958; Prugh, 1953), it was known that the acute responses of a child, especially of a preschool child, to the sudden isolation and desertion of hospitalization caused depression and withdrawal. This led to a revolution in family access to children in hospitals. Having a parent or parent surrogate around most, if not all the time, allowing parents full access to their children, and allowing children access to play rooms and opportunities to play out their problems, even in the days before the onrush of technical medicine began to make families an important component of the treatment of the child in the hospital. Over the past 15 years, there has been an attempt to change the parent from a passive observer to an active therapeutic tool, since the needs of modern medicine virtually dictate a greater level of involvement than was formerly necessary. Some of the studies that we will summarize below indicate that children benefit

more from that type of approach than from one in which child and
family are passive recipients of the mysteries of modern medicine
from an autocratic system.

Fifteen years ago, there was a growing recognition that highly
specialized approaches and highly specialized hospitals were being
organized to provide care for children with exceedingly complex and
difficult disorders requiring major surgery of a type that had
hardly been contemplated before the 1960s. The growth of tertiary
care medicine has drawn a great deal of interest not only from this
author, but also investigators such as Prugh (1953), Mattsson (1973),
and a number of other child psychiatrists who recognized that
approaches to families and children would require significant
changes. Our attention was drawn to the problem by the accidental
finding of significantly acute catastrophic and disorganizing
psychological reactions on the part of children, adolescents, and
young adults in the highly unusual setting of the National Heart
Institute.

Because of the occurrence of these reactions, an effort was
made to study a large group of children and families who were at
first evaluated as "normal" referrals. These families and children
often came from all parts of the United States and the world, from
all types of backgrounds. The purpose of this study was to define
how children responded to major surgery. This study followed an
earlier one (Danilowicz and Gabriel, 1971), where we found that some
of the problems in recovery rooms and ICUs led to psychoses, a
finding observed by other researchers as well (Kornfeld, 1965). The
families that were studied had little or no opportunity for
preparation prior to the surgery. In general, the families were
passive participants in the care of their children, or, in fact,
sometimes were not available for long periods of time. The kinds
of responses that occurred with normal children during their
hospitalization are categorized in Table 1.

Some of the abnormal responses noted in Table 1 will be
addressed later. On the basis of this initial data, we attempted
to find ways to mitigate short-term responses, with the hope that
minimized short-term responses might result in minimized long-term
psychological responses.

Based on this study of psychoses and childrens' responses to
the tertiary setting, an awareness arose that families were often
as helpless and confused as their children, and that some of the
earlier techniques of vaguely acqua nting families and children
with a "trip to the hospital" or play with dolls in the hospital
did nothing to help mitigate the reactions to the new technology.
Furthermore, it seemed that the new major techniques required a
new level of cooperation by both child and parents and a tolerance

of discomfort that may not have formerly existed. For example, it is essential that children having major surgery not be sedated to the point where they cannot cooperate with pulmonary exercises and coughing procedures, which prevent post-operative complications following chest surgery. This is also true of such surgery as amputations, reimplantations, plastic revisions and abdominal surgery. However, with the analgesic medicines that are available, the discomfort can and should be moderated. In addition, the vast array of new machines and methods in cardiac catheterization laboratories, recovery rooms, intensive care units, and even wards, tends to create concern and confusion regardless of the type of surgical procedure.

There are two issues that relate a bit more specifically to open-heart operations than to other surgical procedures in tertiary care hospitals. The first is the special symbolism of the heart, and what it represents to parents, and, indeed, to older children. The second, while not unique to cardiac surgery, is more common than in other major operations. This is the phenomenon of operating on an asymptomatic child. A significant percentage of children coming to elective cardiac surgery are referred because a murmur is heard, and laboratory evaluation has confirmed the presence of an operable lesion. Since the child may be asymptomatic and is not considered ill by the family, compliance with the physician may become a problem.

Our initial studies indicated that several aspects of the hospitalization and surgery had not been integrated by either families or children. This lack of integration was a significant barrier to adjustment. It was then necessary to define for each family the reality they would be exposed to within the hospital setting. While this principle appears obvious, implementing it is harder than one thinks. It would seem that, since development consists of many exposures to many realities on an incremental basis, such a concept is obvious. Nonetheless, families and professionals, responding to their own need to maintain control, often attempt to insulate patients from the "trauma" of reality, and initially tend to resist such a concept. Therefore, it became one of our original tasks to show that families and patients were more cooperative and manageable when allowed to enter into the care system. This, then, led to a protocol that diminished the use of play situations as preparation, and increased the use of reality as a method of introduction to the hospital. It became the physician's responsibility to educate the family not only to the issues around surgery, but also to the hospital milieu. An additional need was to establish with the family a basis for truthfulness between the preparer (physician) and the patient. This meant that the physician had access to the patient after informing the family of the need for orientation and visitation prior to catheterization and/or surgery.

The patient would, therefore, be prepared with the family's collaboration and the physician's active participation. This would first
take the form of verbal communication and sometimes the use of a
heart model in the cardiologist's office, and a visit to the hospital itself prior to the actual hospitalization. The family is informed and must give permission to allow the patient and themselves
to be taken to those areas of the hospital in which the child is expected to be a conscious participant in the efforts of the professional staff. For example, a child who comes in for cardiac catheterization prior to surgery would visit the ward where a nurse would
show the child a typical room, the various play areas, and introduce
the child to a number of the personnel on the ward. The child with
the family is then taken to the cardiac catheterization laboratory
where, rather than playing with toys, the child is allowed to role-
play the cardiac catheterization with a trained member of the
catheterization laboratory staff. This includes "learning" how the
machines work, trying out certain of the techniques, and being told
truthfully when and how needles would be given and what procedures
would be done. This was done with every child over the age of three,
since that is the age when communication becomes possible. Younger
children, if precocious, were also allowed this opportunity. This
technique of preparation has resulted in better cooperation with less
sedation needed during the procedure and, perhaps, with a lowering
of morbidity. With such a baseline condition, the results of an
examination such as the cardiac catheterization would be more valid.

Prior preparation also allowed families to feel less anxious
about the mysteries of the techniques involved for children who then
went home to come back later rather than coming directly into the
hospital for surgery. This allowed for a certain amount of positive
transference to the hospital and personnel. This made the second
visit in preparation for surgery run more smoothly. Unfortunately,
this ideal is not always possible in all cases in a tertiary care
setting. If the child was catheterized elsewhere, the preparation
for surgery was similar except that the ICU and recovery room were
visited and trained personnel would provide instruction and exposure to those situations in which the child and family would be
significantly involved while in a conscious state. Families were
not taken to the operating room, since induction anesthesia was used
prior to moving into that area, and it seemed unnecessary to require that exposure. It was only after these exposures to reality
issues that play and talking (when warranted) by both the families
and the workers who were involved with these children were encouraged.
The results of our follow-up study are summarized below. However,
some of the practical problems deserve further attention at this
point.

The sequence of involvement by the helping professional was always an issue, and it was clear that there might be initial resistance on the part of families with younger children to exposure to

the hospital scene. It was felt, however, that in the face of adamant refusal of preparation of the child, families would be confronted with the possibility of not having the surgery done or having it done elsewhere if they were unable to make a minimal collaborative effort. In fact, only one family out of more than 150 over the years ever had to be confronted with this choice. However, even under ideal circumstances, children's responses to the pain and difficulty of adapting to all the complexities of the hospital resulted in some regressive and difficult behavior (see Table 1). Our effort was to minimize the pain, but not fool ourselves into thinking that the entire hospitalization would go smoothly and not present some difficulties. Even the best preparation cannot cover the tremendous variety of experiences the child and family will encounter during the two-week hospitalization. The scope of the problem was presented in a survey done at the National Children's Hospital in Washington, D.C., indicating that the average child coming in for major surgery will meet more than 70 strangers doing mysterious things during the first 24 hours of hospitalization. Reality preparation added a new dimension of family involvement in immediate post-operative management and care by having them expect certain types of behavior from the children. Parents were encouraged to stay full time, either on a rotating basis or together, and sleeping provisions were made for them. The cardiologist was expected to indicate what they would have to tolerate from the child in the way of irritability, anger, and, to some extent, withdrawal. They were helped to understand some of the dynamics of these behaviors so that they could actively reassure the youngster during the most difficult periods. While it was not possible to predict in any given child to what degree regression would take place or how it would express itself, parents were counseled to expect some sleep disturbances, some regressive behavior such as enuresis and nightmares (especially in the younger child), and were also counseled to expect some of these behavioral responses to continue for a period of time after discharge from the hospital.

A group of 50 parents and children were studied at New York University for short- and long-term sequelae following cardiac surgery (Gabriel and Danilowicz, 1978). The period of follow-up varied from six months to four years. To summarize, it appeared that short-term responses of a gross nature were minimized, except in one child who had serious medical complications and required more than two months in the hospital, much of that time spent in an ICU. Most regressive behavioral responses occurred in the children aged two to seven, and disappeared by one to two months after the operation. Half of these children had nightmares, restless sleep, difficulty falling asleep without a parent in the room, wanted to sleep with the parents, and returned to the need for a security object or light. Almost all of these reactions subsided within two to four weeks, with the exception of the child with the complicated, prolonged hospitalization mentioned above, who took a year to recover. This five year old child

Table 1. "Normal" Postoperative Reactions in Children Undergoing Cardiac Operations (N=61)*

Item	Reaction			
	Anxiety (N=28)	Cooperation (N=16)	Anger (N=10)	Compliance (N=7)
Operation				
Thoracotomy	13	2	1	2
Open-heart	15	14	9	5
Medical complications				
4	2	0	0	0
3	4	2	6	0
2	8	3	0	4
1	4	7	3	3
0	10	4	1	0
Average number of days in intensive care room	2.0	2.6	2.8	1.7
Average age	6 years 4 months	10 years 9 months	10 years 3 months	10 years 1 month
Age range (in years)	1.5-11.5	5.7-15.6	6-14.7	6.8-15

*Not included are four children who had abnormal reactions, two infants, and a child who died without regaining consciousness

Since we were able to note their reactions, two children who died three days and five days after their operations are included

regressed to the bottle and could not separate from her mother. Almost all other children had a great need to review the hospitalization verbally many times over with the parents and other family members or friends. They involved themselves in certain counter-phobic behaviors, such as showing off their scars to all comers and regaling them with the events of the hospitalization. Interestingly enough, the child with the complicated long-term course entered this phase about a year later, and made a rapid recovery after that without psychiatric intervention. On the other hand, adolescents seem not to be as verbal or as counter-phobic as younger children, but our sample was not large enough to make clear conclusions as to how adolescents integrate their hospital experience on a long-term basis. No children in this small group appeared to have any problems in the immediate post-operative period, and none showed serious adjustment problems. By and large, the reactions following the approach described appear to be relatively mild, although a few trends appear that slowed the process of post-hospitalization integration. Those families which appeared to be repressing and denying in nature slowed the post-operative adaptation period and on occasion other hospital personnel would be utilized to encourage verbalization. There were not enough of these families in our group to make a definitive statement, but if identified, such families probably would need extra work and counseling. There appears to be no doubt that children who have long, complicated hospitalizations or children from disturbed families run the risk of more complicated psychological courses.

One of the issues most relevant to us is how to identify disturbed families in a fashion that would be simple enough to be useful to the primary care physician, pediatric cardiologist or cardiac sugreon. From the studies of "control" cases, that is, patients managed differently than already described by other groups both within our setting or at the National Heart Institute, only a few clues emerge. Families that are unable to allow themselves or the physician to realistically deal with the issues involved seem to run a clear risk of increasing the negative responses in the hospitalized child. One such example was a child at the National Heart Institute who had the following experience:

Ann, a five year old white girl, was referred to the NHI for closure of a ventricular septal defect. She was first hospitalized for catheterization, which she handled well, although she was somewhat infantile for her age, sucking her fingers during times of anxiety. In spite of instructions to the parents about preparation, this was not done and the child was told she was coming only for a clinic visit at the time of admission for operation. Her reaction to everyone preoperatively was one of pure, unmitigated fury. The operation was uncomplicated, but afterward the child withdrew from all contact. Ann refused feedings, screamed and lashed out at anyone who touched her. When left alone, she assumed a fetal position in the middle of the bed with her eyes closed, sucking her fingers. She became incontinent of feces and urine. By the end of the first week her fingers were raw and bleeding. Nasogastric feeding was required and the parents were totally ignored by the child when they visited. Because of her inactivity, the child developed atelectasis and secondary pneumonia. Since nothing seemed to help, the child was given a specific date of discharge and within 48 hours, she began to eat, watch television and interact with the nurses. She became continent and the pneumonia quickly cleared. Although the atelectasis was still present, she was discharged as promised and the lungs were clear on her first post-operative visit. Although superficially the anger had subsided, the child acted out at home for almost one year. Her return visit to clinic, because of the previous lie, was highlighted by screaming and kicking until she was finally convinced that she was not going to stay.

This girl dramatically shows a possible response in the unprepared and deceived child. Ideally, once the situation was recognized, it would have been better to postpone the operation and reschedule it after proper preparation. This was not done, however, and, as a consequence, everyone suffered. In spite of what appeared to be psychotic withdrawal, this child was in excellent contact throughout. She recited in detail everything that occurred during this episode, and the dramatic results after being told of her discharge date confirm this. It is quite likely that even after the overt acting out was over, this child's parental distrust continued to manifest itself in other personality traits.

Another type of family that seemed to run increased risks are rural, foreign, or new immigrant families who are considerably less sophisticated than urban middle class families. Such a problem is exemplified by the following case:

Bob, a 15 year old non-English speaking Greek boy, was referred to the NHI for re-operation for mitral insufficiency. A prosthetic mitral valve had previously been placed, but breakdown of the suture line resulted in recurrence of congestive heart failure. During the early portion of his hospitalization, he was anxious but friendly and bright. After catheterization and before his operation, Bob wrote several short stories concerning death in young boys and men. Operative repair of the suture line required minimal pump time but insertion of a pacemaker was required for the first twenty-four hours to control arrhythmias. On the fourth day in the intensive care room, he became agitated and could not be restrained in bed. Bob insisted that his valve had come out and that he had to find it or he would die. He looked in the bed sheets, under the bed and around the room. He would not listen to reason, appeared

to be out of contact, and was finally given intramuscular sedation. About six hours later, Bob was back in contact and had
little memory of the event. He was discharged to the ward the
following day and the remainder of his hospital stay was un-
eventful.

It is likely that the added isolation consequent to the language problem increased the likelihood of a psychotic break in this
boy. The need for two major procedures in a relatively short time,
combined with the arrhythmia post-operatively certainly increased
the level of anxiety. Because of the arrhythmia, Bob was kept on
monitor in the intensive care room for a longer time than usual and
this environment probably contributed to the reaction. A letter from
the family in Greece about one year later indicated that the boy was
back in school and doing well. No mention of any problems was made.

We have used these two cases to exemplify the kinds of issues
that can be directly preventable rather than describing the complexities of families and children with prior psychopathology. These
latter problems require special handling and involvement of psychiatric personnel, and usually represent, with one exception, a very
small proportion of children coming to major surgery. The one general exception is that of the retarded child who can be handled in much
the same way as the normal child, provided communication is possible.
Nonetheless, families with a retarded child represent a specific type
of problem since they are burdened with guilt and some divisiveness
around the care of the child as a result of mental disability. We
have had experience with several cases in which the parents were of
such differing views that even the question of surgery took a long
time to resolve. Certainly, it is true that an initial careful history can often identify preexisting family disorganization that might
be expected to result in child psychopathology, and this we urge be
done for every patient who needs to be exposed to complex surgical
intervention.

A final word about the world we live in regarding the modern
hospital: A significant part of the evolution of the techniques
described earlier was based on some of the difficult realities we
all face in our current culture. The growth of the PSRO, the need
to get what has to be done done quickly now makes it virtually impossible to prepare a child adequately when he first arrives at the
hospital. It is all too common for a child to be admitted on Sunday and be in an operating room by 8:00 A.M. the next morning, experiencing a whole new world of complexity and potential distress.
Under these circumstances, professionals must prepare the family and
the patient earlier on an outpatient basis. The fact that staffs
are far too harried within the modern hospital today mandates active
involvement of parents in the care of their children, despite the
inherent reluctance of hospital staffs to deal with the demands of
concerned families. We must all be cognizant that while ideal

theories and ideal understanding may lead to ideal plans, we must all live in a reality that rarely if ever allows these ideals to be achieved.

Summary

This paper presents a number of techniques designed to minimize the psychological problems associated with hospitalization, major open heart surgery, and associated long-terms sequelae in a tertiary care setting. After several preliminary studies, a protocol for pre-hospital preparation and a plan for hospital management were designed. The plan was designed to be used by pediatric and nursing staff in a tertiary care pediatric setting. The initial goal was simply to minimize the incidence of ICU psychoses and other serious post-operative behavioral responses in the hospital. Follow-up studies after discharge were done, and indicated that most patients had minimal post-hospitalization psychological difficulties. Overall, children in the age group from 3-6 had somewhat more adjustment problems after hospitalization than children who were either younger or older than that age group. Regression to more infantile levels of behavior for several months was most commonly noted. Out of the group of 50, only one child, who had an extended hospitalization showed any serious psychopathology. This reaction diminished during the course of one year. Several cases of children who had severe reactions in the hospital probably consequent to inadequate preparation are also discussed.

REFERENCES

Bowlby, J. Separation anxiety. International Journal of Psycho-Analysis, 1960, 41:89-113.

Danilowicz, D.A. & Gabriel, H.P. Postoperative reactions in children. 'Normal' and abnormal responses after cardiac surgery. American Jrnl of Psychiatry, 1971, 128:185-188.

Danilowicz, D.A. & Gabriel, H.P. Post-cardiotomy psychosis in non-English speaking patients. Psychiatry in Medicine, 1971, 2:314-320.

Danilowicz, D.A. & Gabriel, H.P. The response of children to cardiac surgery. In Modern Perspectives in Psychiatry Series, Brunner/Mazel, New York, New York, 1976, pp. 267-284.

Gabriel, H.P. & Danilowicz, D.A. Postoperative responses in the 'prepared' child after cardiac surgery. British Heart Jrnl, 1978, Volume XL, No. 9, pp. 1046-1951.

Kronfeld, A.A., Zimberg, S. & Malm, J.R. Psychiatric complications of open heart surgery. New England Jrnl of Medicine, 1965, 273:287.

Naylor, K. & Mattsson, A. For the sake of the children; trials and tribulations of child psychiatry liaison service. Psychiatry in Medicine, 1973, 4:389-402.

Prugh, D.C., Staub, E., Sands, H.H., Kirschenbaum, R.M. & Lenihan, E.A. A study of the emotional reactions of children and families to hospitalization and illness. American Journal of Orthopsychiatry, 1953, 23:70-106.

Robertson, J. Young Children in Hospital. Basic Books, New York, New York, 1958.

Spitz, R.A. Hospitalism: An inquiry into the genesis of psychiatric conditions in early childhood. Psychoanalytic Study of the Child, 1945, 1:130-153.

"To Prepare a Child" (Movie), Children's Hospital National Medical Center, Washington, DC, August 19, 1976.

...

HELPING THE CHILD AND FAMILY WITH SURGERY: DISCUSSION OF

DR. GABRIEL'S AND DR. DANILOWICZ'S PAPER

Irving N. Berlin, M.D.

University of New Mexico School of Medicine

Albuquerque, New Mexico

It is a pleasure to discuss such a clear and straightforward approach to a problem so many of us have found so difficult. Drs. Gabriel and Danilowicz are probably in more fortunate circumstances than many of us who have tried to get both hospital administrators and pediatric and orthopedic sugreons to recognize the importance of family access to children and to provide for overnight stay. In a recent discussion between Dane Prugh and the past President of the Academy of Pediatrics, they agreed that no more than 10% of hospitals serving children either recognize or provide for family access to children.

Similarly, although the authors do not describe in any detail the work they did with their colleagues in Pediatric Cardiology to bring about such an effective procedure, I am sure it took an inordinate amount of skill, tact and persistence to elicit such acceptance.

I have worked in liaison in a Pediatric Department where the Chief had spent many years exposed to Emma Plank's (1971) efforts with children prior to and after surgical procedures. We, therefore, had "Play Ladies" on our wards and some parental access. However it was still very difficult to involve the Pediatric Cardiologist in preparatory work with the parents and child. We simply acknowledged that it might be difficult to help some of our colleagues to become prevention oriented. Thus we circumvented them and members of the Mental Health liaison team; a child psychiatric nurse did much of the preparation and some followup. In retrospect, I wish very much we had knowledge of the authors' work so that we could have done a better job.

There is an elegant simplicity in having the pediatric cardiologist recognize the importance of a very clear, straight-forward
and factual approach to the cardiac catheterization and the surgery which is presented to both the child and parents. The emphasis of the impact on the tertiary care of an automated, multi-
wired and hosed I.C.U. on both child and parent after surgery is
critical. Making the parent a working partner during the recovery
process is an extremely important preventative mental health measure for both parents and child. It seems clear from this paper
that there is a major difference in watching Star Wars on the screen
and being forced to face living with an automated, impersonal group
of robots in the I.C.U. The requirement that the child be able to
tolerate the monitoring machines for optimal results needs re-em-
phasis.

The use of a reality exposure by the physician of the child
and family to the places, machines, etc. that the child will have to
endure and the parents to understand, is indeed the crux of the
authors' preventative intervention. Efforts to explain the disorder, to demonstrate both how catheterization and the surgery was
actually to be done, are clearly a vital part of the reality based
preparation.

I would emphasize that an awareness of the degree of anxiety
in the child and family after such a realistic demonstration would
be an indication that some further work in play therapy with the
child and further discussion with the family by a mental health
professional seems in order. In our experience with a youngster
who had had two previous open-heart procedures, we had to spend
over two months and four play sessions carving on the heart of a
clay figure trying to still the cardiac murmur. Each time the child
died in the pretend surgery. In each session, the high level of
anxiety and the expectable fear of having another surgery was
talked about at length. Only in the fourth play session did the
youngster perform a successful operation on his clay patient. He
performed the same successful surgery two more times prior to hospitalization. This child, terribly apprehensive from his previous
procedures, was gradually able to master the situation and was only
minimally anxious before and after his surgery.

The fact that the procedures, the pain, and the I.C.U. as a
threatening place cannot be totally dealt with, is a reality. The
authors have made clear that that reality must also be anticipated
and talked about. To help parents understand how and why their
child may behave after procedures is very important anticipatory
guidance, which is all too often neglected in the physician's need
to minimize the family's anxieties. The child's temporary rejection of the parents, anger and depression will occur to some
degree even after preparation. Similar anticipation of regressive

behavior when the child returns home is important to the child's recovery and the parents' ability and comfort in dealing with their child.

The need to anticipate how the non-communicative and non-verbal families will understand and react to such intervention is important. Giving them extra time to learn and providing counseling prior to and after a procedure to their child is clearly indicated.

It is logical that a well prepared child and family using the authors' method will come through the ordeal in better shape. As the authors' data show, they need little, if any, subsequent psychological help.

I want to express my appreciation for this excellent paper.

BIBLIOGRAPHY

Plank, Emma N. Working with Children in Hospitals. Chicago Year Book Medical Publishers, 1971.

ARE TOO MANY "LAYING ON HANDS"?: GENERAL DISCUSSION

Audience Member: Child Psychiatrist

I have a question about the fantasies of children. I have been
interested in children with heart surgery since the time I was a
medical student in St. Louis. In playing with these kids and in
listening to their productions, their fantasies frequently centered
around machinery, machines breaking down, such as washing machines
and refrigerators. The one specific area of interest was the
murmur: grade four murmurs and above created considerable tur-
bulence which the youngsters could really feel. I would like to
hear your comments as to how children perceive the murmur and how
they fantasize about it? Is it a volcano exploding? A machine
breaking down?

Dr. Gabriel

First of all, I think the level of understanding and the content of the fantasies is related to the age and to the stage of development. Younger children have many incredibly frightening
fantasies. In the older ones, we get clear fears of dying, only
partly disguised in their comments, "The machines won't work right";
"I won't get the blood put in right"; "He won't do the valve right."
I can't see any consistent pattern to the fantasies, but we haven't
gone around really trying to collect them. You just get a wide
variety of fantasies and, of course, we don't know if our preparation has distorted some of them. You are right! We have heard all
kinds of frightening reactions from the youngsters.

Dr. Swee: Audience Member, Family Physician

I realize that you are located in a major referral center, but
for those of us who are working in a more local setting, there is a
consideration deserving attention: For instance, in our Neonatal
Unit, where there is a lot of involvement of the families already,
staff make great effort to involve the primary care physician, be
it the pediatrician or the family physician. We deal with the
families immediately after the children leave the special ward and

go to the regular ward and, certainly, after the hospitalization.
That's often an important link in the chain of communication. My
question actually revolves around post hospitalization feedback from
the families themselves. Although you pointed up the decreased
morbidity in the children, what kind of follow-up did you do on the
families? What kind of response did you get from the families about
the usefulness of your procedure?

Dr. Gabriel

We did a careful survey of at least 50 families. Most of the
families, except for one, felt very comforted knowing what was going
to happen to their child, where the child would be, and knowing they
had access to the child. All of the families said that the hardest
and most difficult time was waiting during the surgery. The communication problem is that the surgeon disappears from 7 o'clock
in the morning until 3:30 or 4:00 in the afternoon. He finally comes
out to say that it's done. It would be very nice if some system
existed where there could be communication during the course of the
surgery.

In order to remedy the problem, we have all kinds of fantasies
ourselves, like having two-way radios, but you could hear things
that were harmful to the family too. The cardiologist will very
often try to run up and meet with the family. In our center, the
cardiologist is required to be at the surgery, and he really functions as the primary care physician. Unfortunately, our experience
has been that we have more problems undoing some of the things that
some referring physicians do. Those who are willing to come in and
work with us are wonderful--they have the relationship with the
family already in place and it makes a terrific positive difference.

Dr. Mattsson

Both Paul Gabriel and Irving Berlin talked about the various
aspects of preparing a child for surgery, preparing the family,
having the parents as co-therapists in the preparation. You have
the aspect of preparing the family and the child for what will
happen after surgery. You have the aspect of preparing for possible short-lived and/or long-lived emotional reactions to surgery
and the post-operative period. It gets more and more complicated.
I am not as convinced as Irving Berlin seems to be that you should
talk very much about the possible post-operative emotional problems
with the parents before surgery.

How can the preparation of the family and the child with regard to emotional issues be coordinated with the cardiac team?
There are many pediatric cardiologists and cardiac surgeons who are
more concerned about the immediate survival. They would throw you

out of the ward if you start bringing up emotional issues post-operatively with the parents. I am very challenged by what Irving Berlin said. Here again, who in the mental health team should be involved? Dr. Berlin mentioned that the childlife people are very crucial in preparing family members and children in regard to these issues. Could you say a·bit more about this?

Dr. Irving Berlin

We do prepare children for the short-lived possible responses in the I.C.U. There is a second session a day or two before discharge when we talk about longer term sequelae regarding mild regressive phenomena. But who, when, where, and what is always the problem in a big tertiary care system. Staff resistances, which we put up with all over, are the great problem in liaison psychiatry. They are very difficult to deal with.

Jean Stauffer: Audience Member, Social Worker

I thought I would give you a brief 21 year follow-up. I had open heart surgery at age 5, and am very interested in hearing the kind of attention that is now being given to preparation of the child. I was really lucky that my parents were very attuned to all the emotional implications. They were very at ease with hospitals. I would just second the influence of the ICU. One of my most vivid photographic memories from then is that the ICU was indeed a horrifying experience of being pinned down, tubes coming out of every angle, being under an oxygen tent, being out of touch with people. It was frightening.

Dr. Gabriel

In 1959 you were a pioneer. They were just starting.

Jean Stauffer

One intervention I remember being very helpful to me was that I had a large almost life-size doll which I brought into the operating room with me. When I woke and was out of the ICU, she had a bandage on her chest with a tube coming out of it, the same as mine. One of the most painful things I remember was having my bandage changed. I was able to change my doll's bandage before they changed my bandage, and·it just gave me a little bit of control over a very difficult, painful, frightening situation.

Dr. Paul Gabriel

We allow transitional objects. You think they are very good? Because we have had one or two bad experiences. We always tell the family it ought to be the second best toy, not the first. Somehow

the best things end up in the hospital laundry and disappear forever.
We have had one or two Snoopy and Linus blankets go into the hospital laundry to the detriment of the child's mourning process.

Daniel Sabbath: Audience Member, Medical Student

The entry into cardiac surgery for most children is that the
child knows a pediatric cardiologist, probably from the clinic. The
child comes into the hospital to have his or her history taken by a
third year medical student who will be spending six weeks on pediatrics. This student may then do a physical examination prior to
taking blood. Taking blood is hard because the child's veins are very
little, and it's hard to do. Right away, an intern will come who
is a new person to the child. The intern will probably take the
blood and may help with the physical exam. Then the child will be
examined by a cardiac fellow who will probably follow the child
regularly in the hospital. So we have the cardiac fellow and the
medical student regularly seeing the child for tbe next several days.
In addition, nurses will do other procedures, and the pediatric
cardiologist, whom the child may have known for years at the tertiary
care center, will really not be that involved in the day-to-day
care of the child. Have you been able to reduce the number of
strangers that come to the child every day?

Dr. Gabriel

Yes and no. That's why I said 70 in 24 hours.

Daniel Sabbath

Have you been able to do anything about that?

Dr. Gabriel

Well it's the system's problem. Our system is different. Obviously, these patients are told that a medical student will examine them, the house staff will draw blood, and the cardiac fellow
will see them. Most of these children who were not seen in a
clinic make one or two visits to the private attending's office.
The child and family will be seen by the fellow and the cardiologist several times, and the fellow will do the follow-up. Our
cardiologist sees the patient every day and sometimes twice a day
on the ward service. It's a big fellowship and they are making
rounds all the time. One of the reasons my wife Dr. Danilowicz
(co-author) isn't here now is that she would have to make rounds
with the fellows at 4:00 A.M., and neither she nor they were really
quite prepared to do that! I am convinced that an analysis of the
system is the first thing one must do when entering a new place.
You can see where you can enter into and perhaps alter the
system. It is also necessary to keep track of some of the positive

things that are going on, with a knowledge that there are going to
be negative inputs, no matter what you do. The students on short
rotations will always be there, bad interns once in a while will do
a lousy job drawing blood. You can't prepare everybody for everything. There are some things you do have to leave unsaid, and be
prepared to handle problems and their consequences if they emerge.

Dr. Christ

I have not been impressed that children who are hospitalized
necessarily respond negatively to the large number of staff. Most
youngsters over three rather enjoy the attention as long as a
parent is there. They are hurt psychologically less when a procedure is painful, if they and the parent are adequately prepared.
If, however, there are conflicting orders (e.g. You can get up,
You can't get up), great anxiety results. Clear accurate up-to-
date communication is harder but not impossible with a large staff.
This is where a large staff complicates the life of the child and
his family.

FAMILY SYSTEMS THEORY AND CHRONIC CHILDHOOD ILLNESS: DIABETES

MELLITUS

John Sargent, M.D.

Philadelphia Child Guidance Clinic

Philadelphia, Pennsylvania

INTRODUCTION

Chronic illness in childhood presents many diverse challenges
to the affected child, the family, and the medical care system.
Psychosocial implications of the illness must be recognized and
dealt with in conjunction with requisite physiological treatment.
Coordination of the various helping professionals involved in a
given child's care is essential while working toward improvements
in function for the child and his family. Several authors (Battle,
1975; Gliedman and Roth, 1980; Mattsson, 1972; Pless and Pinkerton,
1975; Straus and Glaser, 1975) have reviewed the needs of the child
with chronic illness and his family and described their approaches
toward effective health care intervention. Although these reports
include many useful guidelines and important suggestions for health
care professionals working with chronically ill children and their
families, they do not present a conceptual framework to organize
professional efforts. This paper will present a theoretical approach
to chronic illness in childhood which stresses the system characteristics of the affected child's family. I will also outline roles
for health care providers which support and enhance the family's
ability to organize itself to meet the special demands of a chronic
illness while maintaining effective function for its members in
other spheres. This outline will draw chiefly upon the work of
Minuchin (1970, 1974, 1975, 1978) and his colleagues (Baker and
Barcai, 1970) with children with Juvenile Onset Diabetes Mellitus
and their families.

Inadequacies of Traditional Formulations of Doctor-Patient Relationships and the Sick Role

In the 1950s, Talcott Parsons (1951, 1958) described elements
he felt to be basic to a therapeutic doctor-patient relationship.
In his view, its chief components are: (1) illness is involuntary
and the ill individual is held to be not responsible for his condition; (2) the sick person is exempted from work, family and other
obligations; (3) the patient is expected by society to do what is
necessary to restore his health; and (4) the patient is expected
to seek and follow competent professional assistance in restoring
his health. Parsons notes that the physician suspends normative
expectations of the patient with respect to nonillness behavior
while he fully expects strict and prompt compliance with illness-
relieving recommendations. Although this formulation accurately
reflects prevalent patient and physician attitudes, expectations, and
behavior, it is especially inappropriate in the case of chronic
physical illness. Purely on the basis of the life-long duration and
unchanging nature of insulin deficiency in a patient with Juvenile
Onset Diabetes Mellitus, it is clear that restoration of "health" is
an impossible goal, and suspension of work or school and familial
obligations are counterproductive. The patient is best viewed as not
responsible for the onset of his illness; however, the implementation
of effective treatment routines is the responsibility of the ill
child and his family.

Medical response to diabetes has long been described as management; adaptation (Gallagher, 1976) and adjustment have been viewed
as reasonable and attainable goals of that management. For the
child, normal processes of growth and development have been considered
generally important in planning treatment and assessing its effectiveness. Authors (Battle, 1975; Garner and Thompson, 1978; Mattsson,
1972; Pless and Pinkerton, 1975; Strauss and Glaser, 1975) have
expressed concern about the effects of a child's illness on his
parents and have described the demands which the illness makes on his
family and upon other elements of the child's social context. Multiple social and behavioral maladjustments have been described in
association with a child's chronic illness such as diabetes (Baker
and Barcai, 1970, Garner and Thompson, 1978). Clearly, a more
complete formulation of potential physician, family and affected
child interaction is necessary, taking into account illness management, reciprocal influences of illness and family on one another,
child development, and appropriate functional goals for the child
and family. The premise of this paper is that such a formulation
is possible, utilizing the concepts and concerns of systemically
based structural family therapy. Ultimately, this formulation should
point toward alterations in training of health care professionals
to deal with chronic illness and include new expectations of
physician and family behavior.

Demands of Diabetes Upon the Family

With the diagnosis of juvenile onset diabetes mellitus, several immediate demands are placed upon the child and his family. The family must note and respond to the initial symptoms of the illness and bring their concern about the child to the attention of a competent physician. The family's threshold for response is challenged because of subtle but unremitting changes in the child's behavior and physical condition including progressive weight loss, increasing thirst and frequency of urination, and frequent fatigue. Their usual manner of organization and action in stressful situations is demonstrated as the child comes to medical care, is diagnosed, and hospitalized for initial stabilization and treatment regimen introduction. In my work with newly diagnosed juvenile diabetics in association with Drs. Rosman, Baker and Noguiera in Philadelphia, we have noted families whose initial response to stress necessitated some delay in seeking medical care while one parent attempted to arouse the spouse's concern or where a family rule required that one parent, in particular, bring the child for evaluation. One embarrassed child concealed sheets that he had wet because of his polyuria which also delayed the diagnosis.

The family must accept the lifelong nature of diabetes and appreciate the illness conceptually. Initial shock upon the diagnosis of chronic illness, together with a form of a grief reaction on the part of the child and his family have been well described (Geist, 1979). The family must manage these emotional responses. The boundary between parents and the ill child is tested as the parents must support and comfort one another while both assist the child in understanding and accepting persistent changes in his usual physical integrity.

During the initial hospitalization, the family must develop an entirely new area of instrumental competence. The following tasks are to be mastered: performing insulin injections; deciding upon insulin dosage; doing, recording, and evaluating urine testing; and becoming familiar with dietary requirements and planning meals in a more regulated time sequence. Time must be re-ordered to include these new tasks in conjunction with increased scrutiny of food intake and urination (Benoliel, 1975). Further, knowledge of the symptoms of hypoglycemia, with the immanence of serious danger, must be developed. As the family becomes competent in carrying out these tasks, they establish the confidence necessary to manage the child's diabetes at home.

The limitations of the scope of disability associated with childhood diabetes, appropriately treated, must be accurately understood both by the affected child and his family. Adequate psychosocial function, continued age appropriate development, and

academic progress are reasonable expectations of a juvenile diabetic.
The family must appreciate and support these expectations.

Concepts of Normal Family Function

Every family develops repetitive and predictable patterns of
interaction to preserve family integrity while enabling family
attempts to achieve goals such as nurturing children, pursuing
economic support, and maintaining the spouse relationship. Through
these interactions, emotional distance between people (and thereby,
alternatively, dependency and autonomy) is regulated, demands of
stressful situations are met, and tasks are allocated and conflicts
resolved. Through potentially supportive relationships, the family
can provide means for members to manage satisfactorily emotional
distress. Competent management of stressful situations, supportive
assistance with emotional distress, and successful conflict resolution all reinforce one another and lead to further effective family
functioning.

Throughout his development, a child is continually challenged
with new tasks to master and new capacities to acquire. The child
also requires a sense of the importance of his contribution to and
participation in the functioning of his family. The cumulative
effect of these processes is mutually reinforcing with clearly
structured task completion leading to improved self-esteem which, in
turn, will lead to attempt further tasks and so on.

The family, especially through hierarchically based parental
authority, can provide both the structure to limit, sanction and
organize their children's development and the emotional support to
encourage and reward their performance. Defining the child and his
contribution as worthwhile for the family and for the larger society
are most effectively carried out on a day-to-day basis through
family interaction (Minuchin, S. and Minuchin, P., 1974). As the
child grows older, emotional distance between parents and children
alters as the child moves from dependency to greater autonomy.
Boundaries between the family and the external environment must
become more permeable as the child grows. Conflicts must then be
resolved more through negotiation rather than through unilateral
pronouncements.

The challenge of juvenile diabetes in the family is to develop
routines which provide for physically adequate management of the
illness in the affected child while maintaining functioning
supportive to all members and psychologically normalizing for the
diabetic child.

Application of Family Systems Model to Maladaptive Responses of Diabetic Children

The early work focused on individual psychosocial maladaptation in juvenile diabetics (Sterky, 1963; Switt, 1967). Baker and Barcai (1970) point up the confusion resulting from these individually oriented one-time investigations which group all juvenile diabetics together. They propose a typology which differentiates among diabetics according to both psychosocial integrity and medical condition. Minuchin (1975, 1978) delineated two distinct groups of poorly adapted and poorly functioning children. As the families of these children were seen together both in a specific stress interview and in the performance of certain standardized tasks, particular patterns of dysfunctional family interaction clustered together with each group of poorly functioning diabetics.

Brittle diabetics. The first group consisted of brittle diabetics who developed repeated and frequent episodes of ketoacidosis but whose diabetes was easily managed in the hospital. No medical reason for this difficulty in diabetic control could be determined. These families understood and carried out the tasks of diabetes management and generally complied with medical recommendations. However, free fatty acid levels (directly related to the development of ketoacidosis in diabetes and a biochemical correlate of stress) were noted to increase in these diabetic children when they were introduced into an interview in which their parents were discussing an area of conflict (Minuchin, 1975, 1978). The management of the child's diabetes is influenced by specific and repetitive patterns of family interaction. Highly enmeshed interactions were noted in association with limited personal autonomy and marked immaturity in the diabetic child. Conflicts among family members were excessively left unresolved and, particularly, conflicts between husband and wife (or parent and grandparent) were expanded routinely to include the diabetic child. As the child became symptomatic, the spouse conflict was submerged or detoured into concern for the child's physical condition. Inappropriate overprotectiveness and excessively rigid and limited family responses to stress were also noted in these families. These families viewed themselves as helpless and incompetent to alter the course of their child's illness and the children had poor self-concepts and felt little sense of control over their lives. When asked to describe themselves, the children responded that they are diabetics first and children second.

The successful treatment of these children and their families through Pediatric-Psychiatric collaboration utilizing structural family therapy resulted in marked reduction in hospitalizations for ketoacidosis and concomitant improvement in age appropriate psychosocial function in the diabetic child (Minuchin, 1978). The goal of the planned interventions is the transformation of the family

into a system which supports the child's age appropriate autonomy,
encourages his competent management of his illness, and addresses
and resolves conflicts successfully. The parents are strongly
expected to decide between themselves what their child must do to
care for his illness and to improve his performance outside the
family. This establishes an effective hierarchy within the family,
while decreasing enmeshment and overprotectiveness. The therapy
requires both inventiveness and the creation of significant intensity
with the induction of a sense of crisis to alter rigid patterns of
conflict avoidance. As the parents discuss among themselves
their differences over managing their diabetic child and reach agreement, they then become more successful in the parental role. The
therapy then supports the resolution of other areas of disagreement, independently, without involving the symptomatic child.
Interactions in the presence of the therapist are utilized to achieve
these goals with the family providing direct evidence to the therapist of their improvement. Clear communication between the therapist
and the pediatrician insures that the latter will also encourage
mutual support between the parents concerning their child's diabetic
management and maintain the parental expectation that the child will
care for his diabetes effectively. The child learns that he will
receive parental support for his ideas and desires, gaining more
control over his illness while reducing the uncertainty of incipient,
uncontrollable ketoacidosis. The child benefits by increased self-
esteem and by increased opportunities to participate with his peer
group in school and activities, leading to improved social ability.

Behavioral diabetics. The second group of diabetic children
with poor medical management and psychosocial adaptation have been
termed "behavioral diabetics" (Baber and Barcai, 1970). These
children were found to be noncompliant with their diabetic treatment
regimens, omitting insulin, failing to follow their diet, etc. Their
families were noted to be poorly organized and ineffective in many
areas. Often, marked parental conflict, either overt or covert, was
apparent. Discipline was ineffective and often inadequate, and
the child's willful and defiant behavior was accepted and accommodated
to by the family. The child disregarded parental directives and
persisted with noncompliant behavior. Some of the families faced
stresses so extreme as to leave little energy available to deal
with diabetic management. These stresses have rendered the family
defeated and unable to cope with illness management. Other families
view their diabetic child as highly vulnerable, requiring extreme
permissiveness. Usual levels of intrafamilial supportiveness, and
clear consistent expectations of the child's behavior were lacking
while the issue of control was left unresolved. Poor diabetic control
can be attention-seeking behavior and is not unlike other forms of
out-of-control childhood behavior. Frequently, one parent was
overinvolved with the child while the other has distant relationships
with both his or her spouse and the diabetic child.

Effective treatment requires active involvement of all family members. Adequate diabetic control is clearly expected and the parents are required to assume authority over their child, mobilizing whatever energy is necessary to accomplish this task. At this point, appropriate diabetic management becomes behavior to be attained in the same fashion as other expected behaviors such as performing chores responsively, attending school regularly, etc. Significant therapeutic direction may be necessary to encourage highly overwhelmed families to pursue this while overinvolved, permissive parents will need support to accept adequately, their child's chronic illness. Direct confrontation is required to alter family patterns of acceptance of their child's misbehavior. Parents who are unable to resolve disagreements concerning appropriate measures to deal with their child's failure to follow his diabetic regimen, must be assisted in that effort by stressing that their child's physical well-being is directly dependent upon their ability to manage his behavior and to enforce his complying with medical treatment. Finally, the parents must support the child in clearly expressing his emotional response to having diabetes.

Governing our pediatric-psychiatric work with both behavioral and psychosomatic diabetic children and their families is an open systems conceptual model:

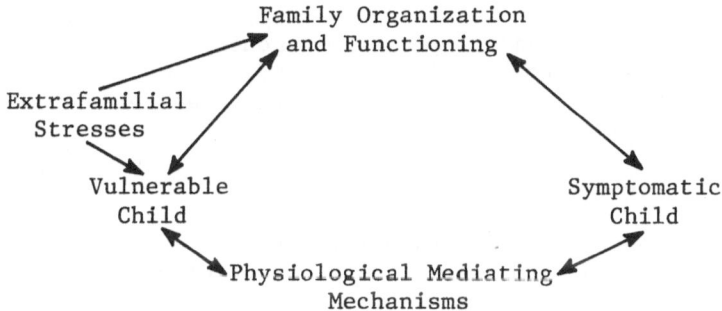

In this model, we find mutual influences among the family, the child, and extrafamilial factors of primary import and that any given element is both caused and causative at any particular time. Extrafamilial factors and features of family organization, which can maintain maladaptive responses in diabetes with poor medical control and psychosocial difficulties, can also be mobilized to achieve good control and functional psychosocial adjustment.

The Effective Family System with Diabetes

What is important for the family is that the management of diabetes be integrated into the usual routines of the family. The illness is a stress like others the family deals with regularly,

like jobs, financial problems, and school for the children. It is
our impression that families who deal with their child's diabetes
as they do other stresses are most successful with the illness.
Mutual support among the parents allows each parent to accept the
illness in their child and deal with the daily potential for medical
difficulty.

     As the parents assist each other, they are then available and
able to assist the child with his reaction to the illness and to
the demands of management. As the parents accept the illness, they
draw on their competence in dealing with previous stresses in
managing diabetes. As they learn, with the child, the tasks needed
for daily illness management, their appreciation of their ability
to cope with the illness is reinforced. As diabetes management
becomes part of the routine of the family, the child can learn that
diabetes is only a part of his life, no more important than its
other aspects. Over time, there can be a reframing for the child
that even with diabetes, he is capable of normal functioning. As
this occurs, age appropriate autonomy is fostered and overprotectiveness becomes less necessary. Finally, with effective support, the
family can competently expect adherence to the diabetic regimen of
the child. In single parent families, these capacities can be
developed by the parent through the utilization of his other support
systems.

     As the child meets family expectations concerning treatment,
self-esteem develops and both family and child can be comfortable
with the child taking responsibility for disease management,
commensurate with his age. This then reinforces, in a feedback
fashion, the child's self-esteem and the family's comfort in maintaining consistent expectations of the child.

     We have also been concerned with the openness of communication
lines in the family and with allocation of roles with respect to
diabetes management among family members. If the child is free
to discuss his concerns about diabetes with both parents, less
misconceptions can develop and his sense of being an intact and
adequate person can be dealt with directly. For parents, role
allocation and open communication go hand-in-hand. If illness
management tasks are divided, constructive communication is essential
for illness related decision making. It is our impression that
flexibility between parents concerning illness management task
performance allows for more effective sharing of the demands of
the illness and more appropriate responses when diabetic difficulties
arise. Sharing to some extent the demands of the illness, the
parents and children can maintain an appropriate boundary which
reduces the possibility of one parent becoming overinvolved with
the child.

     The ability of the family, especially the parents, to resolve effectively conflicts in general and diabetes in particular, is also important in coping with the illness. When to contact the physician? Whether to alter insulin dosage? How to respond to intercurrent illness? How to respond to a child's laxity in carrying out urine tests or adhering to his diet? These are all issues which must be readily and repeatedly negotiated in any family with a diabetic child. The ease with which this is accomplished is directly related to the burden the illness places upon individual family members and the family system. In families with chronic unresolved conflict and power struggles, where each spouse repeatedly takes a position opposing that of the other spouse, the possibility of the child and his illness becoming central issues of family life, is increased.

If, however, mutual support between parents is adequate, parent-child boundaries are appropriate, and conflict resolution is generally successful, there is much less opportunity for the symptoms of the child's diabetes to achieve primacy within the family. Symptoms are easily and effectively dealt with by the child himself when possible. The family organization and level of functioning are not deleteriously affected by the diabetes. The family has the requisite energy to support areas of strength of the diabetic child and to provide for the effective development and individuation of other children in the family. Finally, as the diabetic child learns that his contribution to family life through other aspects of his life remain important, there is a diminishing tendency to utilize his illness for secondary gain and to protect his family from the stresses of diabetes through inappropriate denial.

Implications for Health Professionals

Medical training traditionally emphasizes processes of medical diagnosis and treatment. When interpersonal skills are taught via direct supervision, the major focus is on interviewing, which is chiefly a content oriented, information gathering exercise. More innovative programs now utilize video tape recordings to provide direct access to the trainee's style, but even there, the focus is limited. Recently, structured education materials and programs have been made available to families with a chronically ill member. For diabetes, there are now excellent instructional materials and many diabetes clinics now employ Diabetes Educators--nurses or other professionals trained in providing instruction in disease management tasks. There is, however, no consistent agreement about who is to receive education and this varies from family to family. Physicians also are not taught how to present the diagnosis initially to the family or to assist them in their immediate emotional response. Furthermore, physicians are not provided ways of reinforcing normal adaptation through the course of the illness, nor methods of addressing difficulties which arise.

The approach advocated by this author suggests that the above description of effective functioning and appropriate family coping with a chronic illness, points toward a clear, powerful role for the physician, providing him with various intervention skills and straightforward goals. This approach must build upon a solid knowledge of human pathophysiology and effective physical treatment. The physician must be confident in his recommended treatment and convinced of its appropriateness for a particular patient. For diabetes, general issues of medical treatment are agreed upon and available to most conscientious practitioners. Where there is disagreement among members of the medical community (in diabetes treatment, this includes tightness of control, strictness of diet, etc.), the physician can present areas of controversy to allow the family to decide upon a course of action. He could also decide upon a particular regimen and recommend it strongly, recognizing that the family may choose to disregard his treatment. As the physician goes through this process with a family, he models effective limit setting and appropriate negotiation, which the family can integrate into their interaction with the diabetic child.

The physician also must deal with his own feelings concerning the uncontrollable incidence of a serious chronic illness such as diabetes. He must accept his own powerlessness to prevent the illness while maintaining confidence concerning normalized psychosocial adaptation and function-reinforcing medical treatment. This recognition allows the physician to appreciate both the initial emotional reactions to the diagnosis by family members while modeling effective coping.

We strongly advocate education of all family members in the household and significant caretakers in concepts of diabetes and its management. At the close of the education sessions, the family is required to demonstrate competence in the tasks of management and in deciding how to respond in difficult situations, e.g., emergence of hypoglycemia, intercurrent infection. By demonstrating their knowledge, the family can receive praise for their efforts and be provided any necessary further instruction. The physician should expect the family to be reasonably confident in their ability to carry out the daily routine while understanding how to receive medical assistance when necessary.

Information about family structure, overall family function, and the family's patterns of adaptation to stress and change is provided the physician during the education process and meetings with the family concerning diagnosis. This information can enable the physician to develop hypotheses concerning the family's adequacy of adaptation to diabetes. The physician's task is then to encourage flexibility and mutual support among family members. The physician's confidence will enable the family to make necessary realignments of schedules and priorities. This process is abetted by the physician delineating the family's previously demonstrated capacities of organization and effective parenting. He will need to learn how to search for family strengths and to reframe situations so as to point out to family members their abilities to manage successfully the diabetes at home. This is especially true during times when family members become overwhelmed by the complexity of disease management.

Physicians also must become experienced in the role of consultant to the family, as well as director of treatment. This will include questioning family members at regular intervals about who performs illness related tasks and how illness related decisions are reached. Physicians are trained to answer questions, but now they must learn to stimulate family members to develop answers among themselves to their questions. This further encourages increased cooperativeness and supportiveness within the family. By determining how successful the parents are at ensuring routine disease management, the physician can also support and strengthen parental executive function when required.

Family meetings can be scheduled, if necessary, to provide the family with a forum for resolving disagreements concerning illness management. The physician can also support more effective task allocation. Furthermore, intermittent family meetings can serve to determine and strengthen the customary less active role of the father in diabetic care, his relationship with the diabetic child, and his support of other aspects of his child's life.

The physician can utilize distribution of diabetes management tasks to emphasize the family's appreciation of the affected child's development and individual autonomy. For younger children, less than eight years of age, the family should be instructed to include the child in urine testing and in preparation for insulin injections. As the child grows older, the physician needs to encourage the parents to allow the child to take more responsibility for the diabetes management, including keeping records and administering insulin. As the physician recommends that the family expedite this process, he is in fact supporting the family's efforts at maintaining age appropriate development. Diabetes management also can provide the child with opportunities for developing increasingly competent self-control with parental reinforcement and praise.

The child's immature behavior, social withdrawal, and excessive dependency upon the parents can never be excused by the physician as in any way acceptable in diabetics. The physician must challenge parental accommodation to immaturity and dependency and assist the family in developing plans to change these behaviors. In order to counter the overinvolvement of one parent with the ill child, which leads to the persistence of immature behavior, the physician will

need to involve actively, the more peripheral parent. This may
necessitate phone calls to the less involved parent, family meetings,
and other forms of direct contact. During this process, the physician
will need to encourage that parent to convince the overinvolved
parent to change expectations for the child.

In order for these interventions to be successful, the physician
will need to be comfortable with giving directives to the family.
Usually physicians are comfortable giving instructions concerning
medication. The knowledge that how families organize themselves
influences the course of chronic illness will enable physicians to
do this confidently. Furthermore, the physician can maximize
successful adaptation by encouraging negotiation between parents
and children about both illness management and other aspects of the
diabetic child's life. The doctor can note and challenge situations
in which parents or relatives undermine each other or maintain
inappropriate reactions to the ill child. This will, of necessity,
include establishing an atmosphere in which the family recognizes
that effective diabetes management and child rearing go hand-in-hand
and are both the responsibility of the parents, with the physician
providing suggestions and support.

CONCLUSION

I am proposing that physicians recognize that the locus of
control of a chronic illness such as diabetes resides within the
family. This approach requires a basic change in approach toward
provision of medical care in chronic illness. It expects that
physicians will be competent medically, share this competence with
family members, and support improvements in self-esteem which arise
from successful management of the crisis of diagnosis and integration
of illness related tasks into daily life. It is based upon a
coherent theory of family functioning against which the physician
can judge any family's current effectiveness. The approach also
expands the physician's alternatives for intervention at any point
in the course of a chronic illness, while directly amplifying his
power in problem situations. The physician can clearly note
difficulties developing, address them early in their course, and
move rapidly the direction of successful family adaptation.

Finally, this approach will require that the physician develop
additional interpersonal skills and significant confidence in
utilizing them. The reward for this effort, beyond increased options
for providing effective medical care, will be a deeper sense of
respect for people's ability to cope with stress, and to foster
development and growth in the face of illness.

REFERENCES

Baker, L. and Barcai, A. Psychosomatic Aspects of Diabetes Mellitus.

In: O. W. Hill (Ed.) Modern Trends in Psychosomatic Medicine, Vol. 2, New York: Appleton-Century-Crotts, 1970.

Battle, C. U. Chronic Physical Disease--Behavioral Aspects. Pediatric Clinics of North America, 22:525, 1975.

Benoliel, T. Q. Childhood Diabetes: The Commonplace in Living Becomes Uncommon. In: A. L. Strauss and B. G. Blaser (Eds.) Chronic Illness and the Quality of Life. St. Louis: C. V. Mosby, 1975.

Gallagher, E. B. Lines of Reconstruction and Extension in the Parsonian Sociology of Illness. Social Science and Medicine, 10, 207, 1976.

Garner, A. M. and Thompson, C. W. Juvenile Diabetes. In: P. R. Magrab (Ed.) Psychological Management of Pediatric Problems, Vol. 1, Baltimore: University Park Press, 1978.

Geist, R. A. Onset of Chronic Illness in Children and Adolescents: Psychotherapeutic and Consultative Intervention. Journal of American Orthopsychiatry, 19:4, 1979.

Gliedman, T. and Roth, W. The Unexpected Minority-Handicapped Children in America. New York: Harcourt, Brace, Jovanovich, 1980.

Mattsson, A. Long Term Physical Illness in Childhood: A Challenge to Psychosocial Adaptation. Pediatrics, 50:801, 1972.

Minuchin, S. The Use of an Ecological Framework in the Treatment of a Child. In: E. J. Anthony and C. Koupernik (Eds.) The Child and His Family, New York: John Wiley and Sons, 1970.

Minuchin, S. Families and Family Therapy, Cambridge: Harvard University Press, 1974.

Minuchin, S. and Minuchin, P. The Child in A context: A Systems Approach to Growth and Treatment. In: U. B. Talbot (Ed.) Raising Children in Modern America, Boston: Little, Brown, 1974.

Minuchin, S., Baker, L., Rosman, B. L., Liebman, R., Milman, L, and Todd, T. A Conceptual Model of Psychosomatic Illness in Children. Archives of General Psychiatry, 32: 1031, 1975.

Minuchin, S., Rosman, B. L. and Baker, L. Psychosomatic Families-Anorexia Nervosa in Context. Cambridge: Harvard University Press, 1978.

Parsons, T. The Social System, New York: The Free Press, 1951.

Parsons, T. Definitions of Health and Illness in the Light of American Values and Social Structure. In: E. G. Taco, (Ed.) Patients, Physicians and Illness, New York: The Free Press, 1958.

Pless, I. B. and Pinkerton, P. Chronic Childhood Disorder-Promoting Patterns of Adjustment, Chicago: Yearbook Medical Publishers, 1975.

Rosman, B. L., Minuchin, S., Liebman, R. and Baker, L. Family Therapy for Psychosomatic Children: Follow-up and Outcome. Presented at Meetings of the Academy of Psychosomatic Medicine, November, 1978.

Sterky, G. Family Background and State of Mental Health in a Group of Diabetic School Children, <u>Acta Paediatrica</u>, 25: 1, 1963.

Strauss, A. L. and Glaser, B. G. <u>Chronic Illness and the Quality of Life</u>, St. Louis: C. V. Mosby, 1975.

A USEFUL GUIDE TO FAMILIES WITH JUVENILE DIABETES: DISCUSSION OF

DR. SARGENT'S PAPER

David M. Kaplan, Ph.D.

Stanford University School of Medicine

Palo Alto, California

It is a pleasure to discuss John Sargent's paper, because he offers the health professional a very useful guide to understanding families who are confronted with juvenile diabetes and because he provides a clear basis for some forms of intervention which those families require. The author recommends to us a particular theoretical approach to chronic illness, an approach I find compatible with my own experiences and thinking--and that's pleasing too.

As I interpret Dr. Sargent's theory, he conceives of the family as the "locus of control," as the central mediating system for the stresses generated by chronic illness. He describes family responses to chronic disease as the result of a problem-solving process, and not simply as expressions of individual or collective psychopathology. According to Dr. Sargent, adaptation to chronic illness involves the patient, the family and their physician in a process of interaction and disease management. Parenthetically, I would amend this triad by substituting the health care system for the physician, who participates as a member of that system. Of course, the health care system is more than just the physician--it includes all health professionals, as well as health institutions such as hospitals, clinics, all of which influence families profoundly in their coping efforts.

In his paper, Dr. Sargent outlined the specific problem tasks that must be accomplished if the family is to achieve a realistic accommodation to childhood diabetes. These tasks include: (1) recognizing that the child's initial symptoms require early medical evaluation; (2) accepting the chronic nature of this illness; (3) developing family competences required by the illness; and (4) making appropriate demands for self-care of the ill child.

The author emphasizes the need for open family communication which permits difficult questions to be asked freely, and painful emotions to run their course as part of the process of coming to terms with serious illness. If a family accomplishes these tasks, the chances are good that its members will be able to live without unnecessary distress, disability, or restrictions, and will be able to enjoy satisfying lives despite the existence of chronic illness. If, for any reason, these tasks are not resolved, the family members are likely to suffer from a variety of problems as individuals; they will be members of a family unit that may be permanently weakened in carrying out ongoing mediating responsibilities or destroyed as a result of failing to adapt to the illness.

Dr. Sargent indicates that interventions for families with juvenile diabetes should be guided by the situational task analysis he has described. Interventions should be based upon specific knowledge of what goes into effective coping and mediation with diabetes. He offers "a coherent theory of family functioning against which the physician can judge any family's current effectiveness."

Interventions take several forms including: (1) the education of families and of health professionals in disease management tasks and in the components of effective coping and mediation; (2) the treatment of families who can't cope with the illness on their own; and (3) the treatment of individuals unable to cope independently with the illness. I would add another form of intervention, (4) system intervention aimed at modifying the behavior of health care personnel who either interfere with individual and/or family efforts to cope or who fail to promote healthy adaptation. System modification can include modification of the policies of health institutions. All forms of intervention are integrated by knowledge of the problem-solving process required by each illness.

Throughout the paper, Dr. Sargent refers to the "physician" who takes responsibility for both the physical and psychosocial aspects of chronic care. To me, the term "physician" for diabetes refers to the pediatrician or family doctor who assumes responsibility for the total care of patient and family. I am convinced that most families want "their doctor" to be the one they can turn to for all aspects of care including the interpretation of what "specialists" recommend. Most people resent being farmed out for pieces of their care, e.g. to psychiatrists to handle their psychosocial problems. The approach recommended by Dr. Sargent means there will be less likelihood that patient/family care will be fragmented by "specialists"--and that is an objective worth striving for.

ADOLESCENCE: AN EXTRA HURDLE FOR THE DIABETIC: GENERAL DISCUSSION

Dr. Larry Solter: Audience Member--Psychiatrist

Dr. Sargent, would you comment on children who have had diabetes from ages four to six when they enter adolescence? Is it normal, expected behavior of which the families need to be informed and can therefore anticipate or whether the difficulties usually point to some problem in the family or in the system? In my experience, diabetic children, when they enter adolescence, do run into management difficulty at that time.

Dr. Sargent

You need to make a judgement about the severity of the diffi-culty. Certainly Dr. Mattsson's talk yesterday was illustrative of expected risk taking behavior in adolescent hemophiliacs. One expects that an adolescent with diabetes is going to experiment about the limitations and abilities of his body. It's my feeling that that takes place the same way as experimentation with not doing one's homework, not doing chores, and later on with sexual acting out, drug use, etc. If the family responds to the experimentation in a certain way, it will play itself out. The child will learn, "Damn it, I gotta have my insulin, otherwise I am going to get sick." Or, he will learn that it is a signal that will involve his parents, keep them interested in him, etc., etc. When it becomes a repetitive pattern of maladaptation, intervention is necessary. With every chronic illness, one experiences different responses to it through different developmental phases for the child and for the family. You can't expect that effective adaptation at age five to diabetes necessarily means that maladaptation never comes up as an issue at age 10 or 15.

Dr. L. Najarian: Audience Member--Child Psychiatrist

Dr. Sargent, I have a question along the same lines that you were just answering. I can accept and appreciate the spirit of challenging immaturity and maladaptive behavior. How do you handle this technically? It almost sounds, and I am sure you don't do it,

but it sounds like you tell the youngster, "Kid, we are not gonna
accept that kind of nonsense. You can't do that."

Dr. Sargent

I don't. But I wonder aloud whether the parents are willing to?

Dr. Najarian

I assume before one can do that, it is done in a background of
having established an alliance with the family. Could you comment
on how you establish that alliance? Several other quick questions
are: Have you had any experience with the new machine where the
insulin is managed 24 hours a day? And, what is the effect of the
machine on the system? Also, I have found that kids who have their
diabetic onset after three or four years of age, after object constancy and individuation separation have taken place, and where
there is a sense of wholeness and body intactness that these children
seemed to do a little better. Any clinical experience regarding
that?

Dr. Sargent

I will try and go backwards. You will have to remind me if I
don't answer each of your questions. We are beginning to look at
diabetes in very young children. There is nothing in the literature
except anecdotal responses to an 18 month old with diabetes. My
sense is that families have a lot of difficulties around the very
concrete issues of daily management. But I don't have data on that.

The second thing is I don't personally have any experience with
the pump in diabetes. My feeling is that will get the kid to have
a lot more control, regardless of when he chooses to use it--in the
same way as wearing glasses does. We are just beginning now with
regular blood glucose monitoring through the lance. Fortunately,
it doesn't hurt a lot, and they can check out and readjust their
insulin dosage to get a lot more accurate control.

With respect to the first question: how I would allow for or
encourage the challenge? I do that within the framework: "You guys
(parents) are fine people. You are clearly interested in getting
everything going here and making sure that your child grows up."
I always take the positive side of the ambivalence in developing
an alliance with the family. And then I say, "Well, how come then?"
I don't say it to the kid because I don't believe that I have enough
ties with the kid in the beginning. But I do believe that the
parents have enough ties with the kid that they can develop ways of
expecting functional behavior from him. I also trust that's going
to take place not only in my office, but at home.

Dr. David Karan: Audience Member

It strikes me that the physician or other professional can very easily get drawn into utilizing the parent who automatically looks like the most competent, and overlooking the less involved parent.

Dr. Dorothy Ramsey: Audience Member--Nurse

I have two concerns partly related to Dr. Karan's question. What do you do about informing parents concerning age appropriate developmental tasks? Or do you think that they have that knowledge already? Secondly, do you find that group work for the family helps them in developing coping mechanisms for this situation?

Dr. Christ

When you say group work, do you mean groups of parents?

Dr. Dorothy Ramsey

Yes

Dr. Alisa Barbon: Audience Member--Psychologist

We are studying two families whose diabetic children have been started on the pump with constant insulin infusion. Sometimes, it takes a tremendous amount of restructuring in the beginning because the child has to be monitored constantly. Family dynamics have to be considered because it is an impossible job for one parent to do and other people have to be brought in to help. It takes a tremendous amount of support from the whole team for the family to get the child adjusted to the pump.

Dr. Marshall Mintz: Audience Member--Psychologist

I have worked with the parents of a child who was put on the pump. Two years of work were done with the parents around the child developmental issues, and then the child, who was a very labile diabetic, was put on the pump. The assumption was that if you put the child on the pump before there was a great deal of independence and autonomy, that you would really create a major problematic relationship shift in the family. Despite all the preliminary work done in this case, one of the parents did become very depressed. A lot of the issues that created the labile diabetes were still a function in the marital dyad. It can throw the family system into quite a turmoil if the child is stabilized too quickly. That is one of the complications of the pump.

<u>Dr. Christ</u>

Drs. Barbon and Mintz, the description of your experiences are addressing the questions that were raised. Let us continue this during the panel discussion later on.

PREVENTION OF PSYCHOSOCIAL PROBLEMS IN HEMOPHILIACS

Åke Mattsson, M.D.

New York University Medical Center

New York, New York

At times, psychiatrists have caused themselves an identity crisis by branching out into areas of community problems, national problems, international affairs, poverty, politics and criminality which they are not well qualified to handle. Many of us have met the fate of Dr. Peck, illustrated in the verse entitled "Psychiatrists Beware":

> There was a doctor named Dr. Peck
> Who fell in a well and broke his neck.
> People said he should have known
> To treat the sick and leave the well alone.

When it comes to the area of chronic illness such as hemophilia, the mental health specialist has something to offer the primary care physician, the hematologist, and other health care team members who deal with hemophiliac patients and their families. Hemophilia is not only a familial disease, it also involves all family members. A biopsychosocial viewpoint is required in order to engage the health care team optimally in the care of the hemophiliac patient and his family. The psychosomatic viewpoint includes the individual's psychological reaction to his illness as well as the implications of his illness for his family. The role of the mental health specialist in the comprehensive program for hemophiliacs is by no means limited to those patients who present psychiatric problems. The mental health professional also is essential for the promotion of preventive work with the hemophiliac and his family, in the area of psychosocial functioning. The various levels of prevention in mental health are:

Primary prevention. The emphasis is on preventing psychosocial complications of hemophilia. We rely on early screening of hemophiliac families and early identification of possible psychological and social problems. These are duties of the comprehensive hemophilia care team.

Secondary prevention. This entails the evaluation and treatment of already manifest psychological problems of the hemophiliac and his family. We may see adjustment reactions to the illness and its complications in combination or independently with educational and family problems. Whatever comes first, the organic illness or the psychological problems. both types of disturbances cash in on each other and often aggravate each other.

Tertiary prevention. Serious psychosocial problems may result that require ongoing psychiatric care, including residential treatment placement, long term family therapy, psychotropic medication, and social assistance. Mental health workers should be cautioned about drawing general conclusions about common personality characteristics and problems in hemophiliac patients because the sample of patients referred for psychiatric service is often highly selected. Frequently, hemophiliacs are referred to a psychiatrist as a last resort for patients who show serious management problems or signs of marked emotional disorder.

With reference to primary prevention, we first note that boys with hemophilia do run a higher than average risk of developing adjustment problems. In common with other chronic illnesses, there is a 15% incidence of adjustment problems, as compared to a 7% incidence in children age seven through eighteen. Secondly, we need to identify the main psychosocial stress factors that impact upon the hemophiliac and his family, and understand how these factors interact and often aggravate each other. Thirdly, we want to outline intervention strategies for psychological and social distress of the patients and their families as promptly as possible and to track their course because coping with hemophilia is a life-long ordeal. We have to remind the families and ourselves that the battle is never won.

In terms of biopsychosocial relationships of hemophilia, the open systems model provides a multiple feedback analysis of the biopsychosocial relationships of hemophilia (Figure 1). This model should replace the old linear model of disease process. The open systems model, based upon von Bertalanffy's (1968) general systems theory, allows for a mapping of the many interrelationships of the hemophiliac, which have to be understood in order for us to provide comprehensive prevention and care. Minuchin and his associates (1975) and Agle and Mattsson (1976) have applied the open systems model to the evaluation and treatment of "psychosomatic" children

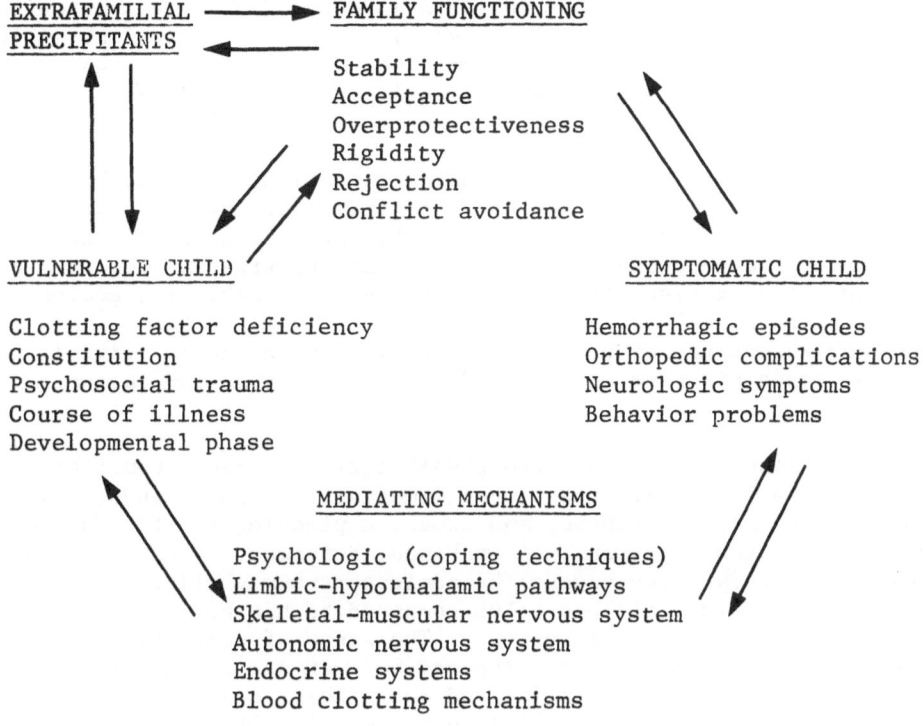

EXTRAFAMILIAL ──────▶ FAMILY FUNCTIONING
PRECIPITANTS ◀──────

        Stability
        Acceptance
        Overprotectiveness
        Rigidity
        Rejection
        Conflict avoidance

VULNERABLE CHILD   SYMPTOMATIC CHILD

Clotting factor deficiency   Hemorrhagic episodes
Constitution   Orthopedic complications
Psychosocial trauma   Neurologic symptoms
Course of illness   Behavior problems
Developmental phase

        MEDIATING MECHANISMS

        Psychologic (coping techniques)
        Limbic-hypothalamic pathways
        Skeletal-muscular nervous system
        Autonomic nervous system
        Endocrine systems
        Blood clotting mechanisms

Figure 1.   Open Systems Model of Childhood Hemophilia

and their families. Certain types of dysfunctional family organization are closely related to the development and maintenance of
psychosocial problems in some hemophiliacs. The patient's illness,
in turn, plays a major role in maintaining the family equilibrium.

Extrafamilial factors pose psychosocial and physical stress
on the family and the vulnerable hemophiliac boy, factors such as
physical trauma, a move, financial burden related to the cost of
medical therapy, reactions by relatives and peers of a belittling,
critical, doting, or unsympathetic nature. Intrafamilial precipitants may be of a physical, traumatic nature, but also of a
psychological nature which stem from maladaptive family functioning
and often impair the hemophiliac's normal development.

The various stress factors impact upon the vulnerable boy--
vulnerable due to his clotting Factor 8 or 9 deficiency. He may
also be vulnerable due to a temperamental constitution, a cyclo-
thymic disposition, or a hyperkinetic trait. The hemophiliac

illness itself, or other physical trauma often add to the patient's
vulnerability in psychosocial terms; impaired intellectual abilities
may result from a cerebral hemorrhage, or severe joint damage
may interfere with normal physical activity, education, and social
relationships.

The developmental phase of adolescence highlights the hemophiliac boy's struggle to achieve a positive, secure sense of self-
esteem. Adolescence is characterized by normal conflicts between
dependence and independence, regressive and progressive forces. A
serious bleeding disorder like hemophilia often makes the adolescent
dependent on health care givers and parents, hampers his social
life and acceptance by peers, interferes with physical activities,
and increases his awareness of having an unreliable and changing
body.

His illness also poses the possibility of serious hemorrhages
and death--all this at an age when immortality, omnipotence, physical
strength and attractiveness, and creative planning for the future
characterize young persons. A weakened, deformed, or unpredictably
functioning body often causes the adolescent hemophiliac to perceive
himself as a person of less value compared to his healthy peers.
This is a blow to his self-esteem. The sense of self-esteem is
based upon the harmony or discrepancy between one's self-representa-
tion (what I know or feel I am) and the wishful self-concept or
ego-ideal (what I wish or feel I ought to be). The hemophiliac
adolescent, more than his younger counterpart, often feels shameful,
depressed, and defective about his body and its functioning. His
self-esteem is low; he is vulnerable to further psychosocial maladaptation as he grows older.

The open systems model includes a set of mediating mechanisms
which, following a hemmorrhagic episode, becomes engaged in the
formation of symptoms, including behavioral problems. Obviously,
the blood clotting mechanisms are essential for the prevention of
hemorrhages.

There are no known direct psychological-CNS influences on the
levels of Factor 8 and 9 in hemophiliacs with low titers of Factors
8 and 9. Starting with the influence of Rasputin on some bleeding
episodes of Tsarewitch Alexis in Russia and continued by dentists
and psychiatrists, there seems to be a set of accumulated empirical
evidence that training in self-relaxation, mild trance or auto-
hypnosis, will reduce the amount of bleeding during dental work
as well as the number of bleeding episodes in certain patients, used
as their own controls, over a period of time. These observations
would be an example of how psychological mechanisms operating within
the hemophiliac's "mind" or CNS, via limbic-hypothalamic pathways
and the autonomic nervous system (ANS), might influence the

peripheral vascular bed via unknown neurohumoral agents. The end
result would be less extravasation through capillary bleeding than
expected in the hemophiliac patient.

The ANS and the vascular bed also relate to the so-called
spontaneous or psychophysiological hemorrhagic episodes. Many
hematologists, parents of hemophiliacs, and hemophiliacs themselves
have described to us that certain states of positive or negative
emotional arousal seem related to an increased bleeding tendency
without clear evidence of physical trauma. The speculative
explanation would be that at times, emotional arousal may, via the
ANS, lead to increased vascular permeability and blood extravasation.
This mechanism would be similar to the one proposed in causing the
painful bruising and ecchymoses seen in patients with psychogenic
purpura and behind the phenomena of religious stigmata.

Many emotional stress factors plague the young hemophiliac,
including bleeding, pain, immobilization, frequent separations from
family, uncertainty about the future, social isolation, and school
absences. What coping techniques are available to the hemophiliac
to deal with his common and recurrent emotional distress? The most
direct or primitive response to physical pain and fears of a
young hemophiliac is the one where his emotional arousal gets
"translated" into physical action, involving the skeletal and neuro-
muscular systems and ANS. These responses include crying, fighting,
and resisting the necessary medical management and physical restrictions. Hopefully, this is only evident in the preschooler,
who still cannot comprehend the cause and effect of his symptoms,
the rationale for shots and other painful procedures, the separation
from his home, and the fact that his loving parents allow strangers
to hurt him. In his egocentrism, the preschool hemophiliac sees
himself as the center of the universe, which means that bad, painful events are caused by him in some way, hence often viewed as
punishment. There are no impartial, natural, and objective
reasons for events, such as an illness, a swollen joint, or a
concentrate infusion even when given by his parents at home. Up
until about age 7, explanations of his condition and of the rationale for treatment won't stick very much due to the boy's pre-
logical, pre-operational thought processes.* Consistent, loving

---

*Stage of pre-operational cognition. Acquisition of language and
symbolic thought: Egocentrism: Everything centers around the child.
Events happen because of him--positive and negative ones. Animism:
Everything is alive, every event occurs by intent. No impartial,
natural causes for events. Magical thinking, words as powerful as
actions. Pre-causal logic: Spatial and temporal juxtapositions
of events. Authoritarian sense of morality--"immanent justice."
Parents always right.

and empathetic reassurance and handling by parents and the medical
staff is the approach essential to the prevention of lasting psychological trauma for children at this stage of development. Child
life programs and hospital based play therapy provide the hemophiliacs a structured outlet for many distressing emotions and
experiences, and mastery through play repetition.

By age seven or so, the hemophiliacs begin to take giant steps
in their cognitive, reasoning thought processes.* Their improved
mastery of words and concepts, their ability to operate in thought
on concrete objects and representations, to group objects and events
like treatment-details and illness-course, and their ability to
understand cause and effect relationships and conceptualize time
better--all these gains are of great help in their coping with
illness. This is illustrated by a seven year old boy who yelled
to his angry mother, "Don't hit me. I'm a hemofishie." The
hemophiliac boys remember, objectively and concretely, what they
have experienced and been told about their symptoms and the treatment. They often begin to report the first signs of a hemorrhage,
cooperate in various treatment procedures, show a beginning
cautiousness in physical play activities, and accept safer, com-
pensatory gadgets and activities. Here, the role of the father and
older brothers can be very helpful.

Repeated, consistent, simple, and understandable explanations,
using drawings and pictures, and time tables related to causes and
treatment of the bleeding disorder begin to pay off for the patient
age seven and older. Ideally, the parents and the health team
should work together, using similar phrases, illustrations, and
realistic reassurances. However, at times of acute bleeding and
other painful events, even the well-adapted seven year old and
older hemophiliacs frequently will show temporary anger, sadness,
and possibly hopeless feelings. This flexible release of natural
distress should be expected by the parents and the medical staff.
The patient's denial of future painful hemorrhages and school
absences does not imply poor reality testing or risk for careless,
dare-devil-like behavior. The grade-school and older hemophiliac
also use such cognitive defense mechanisms as isolation of feelings,

---

*Stage of concrete operational cognition. Logical thought pro-
cesses: Numerical operations; classification; ordering of concrete
object representations. Concept of conservation of reversible
quantities such as size, weight, volume. Exit Santa Claus.
Causality: Logical ordering of events according to chronological,
physical, and psychological factors--past, present, future. Existential awareness. Interpersonal: Can take other's point of view
and communicate with give and take; understands difference between
real and apparent; can reason from premise to conclusion and operate according to rules.

intellectualizations about his illness (control through thinking), rationalizations, and identification with other hemophiliacs and the medical health profession in general.

Adolescence and hemophilia represent a unique combination associated with good psychosocial adaptation or with dangerous states of maladaptation. Ideally, and in most instances, the hemophiliac by then has gained sufficient mastery of his illness and its many stressful factors so the adolescent emotional upheaval will not interfere with his reliable, sensible, self-care and self-protection. After all, most teenagers with severe, chronic illnesses do remain responsible care-takers of their body and good collaborators with the medical team. However, for some adolescent hemophiliacs, the management of their illness gets seriously jeopardized by their poor coping with the major normal tasks of puberty and adolescence.* These tasks are: adjustment to the biological changes with a rise in sexual and aggressive drives and with a reactivation of childhood conflicts with authority figures; achievement of psychosocial independence, a sense of one's own individuality and own identity as a hemophiliac; which requires a loosening of the childhood ties to parents and siblings, often leading to painful states of aloneness and feeling like a stranger amidst the family. States of self-preoccupation and wide mood swings are common, with overevaluation of oneself, alternating with days of self-doubt and self-castigation. What was mentioned before about the frequent, low sense of self-esteem in adolescents with physical deviations, makes them prone to states of depression which might be defended against by daring behavior, rebellious acts, drinking, drug use, eloping, and delinquent acts.

In the area of cognitive development,** the adolescent can

---

*Major tasks of adolescence: (1) Adjustment to biological changes with rise in sexual and aggressive drives. (2) Attainment of psycho-social independence: Development of one's own individuality and sense of identity--"I know who I am"--in relation to peers, family, vocation, and society's expectations and rules. (3) A change in love objects: from parents to extra-familial loving relationships. (4) Development of formal (abstract) thought processes.

**Stage of formal cognitive operations (Metaphysical age par excellence): (1) Combinatorial logic: use of second symbol systems, dealing with many variables at the same time, e.g. algebra, metaphors, ability to "think about thoughts" and to perform. (2) Hypothetical-Deductive reasoning: propositional thinking of "if... then..." type. Construction of systems, theories, ideals, contrary-to-fact situations. Ability to understand, e.g. that if Bob is taller than Joe, and Joe is shorter than Dick, Joe is the shortest of the three. (3) Egocentrism of adolescence: Conceptualizing one's own thoughts and thoughts of others. Preoccupation with one's body,

conduct formal or abstract operational thinking. While usually
assisting him in managing an illness like hemophilia and coopera-
ting with his health-care givers, this gain may at times induce
some hemophiliacs to poor adaptation in adolescence. The ability
"to think about his thoughts," to form theoretical propositions in
a hypothetical-deductive manner,* leads to the special form of
adolescent "egocentrism" which, if overutilized, may turn the
attention of the adolescent hemophiliac to his own body, his own
cognition, and preoccupation with his own emotions in a pathological
way. He may become overly sensitive and self-conscious, seem
parnoid, and experience grave self-doubts and depressive thoughts.
The "imaginary audience" concept refers to the adolescent's normal
tendency to anticipate and imagine the reactions of others to his
appearance and attributes. For example, are they as critical of
the adolescent hemophiliac and his limitations, as he is of himself? The result may be a deepening of his sense of being different
from his healthy peers and feeling isolated. The concept of
"personal fable" refers to the exaggerated belief in one's uniqueness. For example, the hemophiliac may feel he will not get hurt
even if he takes risks because he is invulnerable, immortal, and
specially protected. A stance of "personal fable" often is due
to adolescent egocentrism and rebellious attitudes against parents,
tradition, and compliance with the medical team.

We return to the open systems model (Figure 1) and the impact
of raising a hemophiliac upon the rest of the family. When
learning about his illness, the parents and the older siblings of
a hemophiliac often react with a series of emotions and attitudes.
These may include disbelief, shock, fears and anxiety, anger,
sadness, guilt related to genetic transmission, a sense of helplessness, and finally stoic, realistic resignation and acceptance of
the fate. Family members may reveal the following: father's sadness,
at times, at having produced a defective child; the danger of
antagonism between the parents and the danger of long suffering
martyrdom of the parents; the stress of the healthy siblings of the
hemophiliac, who may experience a lack of parental attention because

---

cognition, emotions, appearance, behavior. "Imaginary audience."
"Personal fable." Normal adolescent "paranoid" stance and prone-
ness to depression. Internal reality. (4) Mature formal operational thinking: After age 15-16. Reconciliation between hypo-
thetical-idealistic theory building and challenge, and realistic
interpretation of experience.

*e.g. "if I receive more cryoprecipate rather than Factor 8 con-
centrates then there may be less risk for liver disease as I get
older, because my doctor has told me all the facts about hepatitis
antigens and liver tests."

of all the care given their sick brother; the problems of a female
sibling, who eventually will be confronted with the fact that she
may be a carrier like her mother. The coping, mastering efforts
of the family members are never over with; that's why we have to
caution against outlining typical sequences of stages of coping
with serious illness.

How does the family organization as a whole (Figure 1) with
its subsystems of adults and children respond to the raising of a
chronically ill child? Ideally, the stable, harmonious family
provides the hemophiliac with a supportive and consistent environment, promoting open discussion about the illness, its management,
and uncertain future courses. All this time, the family shows
respect for the emotional and cognitive developmental state of
the hemophiliac child or adolescent. In marked contrast is the
dysfunctional family whose reaction to a hemophiliac child, or
any different child, jeopardizes his psychosocial adjustment and
normal growth. The first common dysfunctional family type is the
one characterized by overprotectiveness and enmeshment--everyone
is overinvolved and responsive to a sneeze at home, a hollering, a
hemorrhage, a friendship-fallout, etc. This family is prone to
retard the young hemophiliac's development of autonomy, competence,
and responsibility for his own care. The second common type of
family dysfunctioning is the one of rigidity, where change and
personality growth are difficult, not encouraged, and not welcomed.
Neither are new treatment approaches or health providers welcomed.
Rigid parents often cannot accept their son's increased need for
independence, decision-making, choosing of friends and activities--
which may at times be associated with medical risks. The danger
is great that such parents, in their rigid inflexibility, will
precipitate rebellious and risk-taking behavior in their hemophiliac teenager.

A third pathogenic family constellation is the one of overtly
rejecting and negligent parents. This is a rare set, often fright-
ful to observe and difficult to try to change. These are the
parents who have turned their backs towards their hemophiliac son,
partly because of intellectual limitations, and partly because
of long-standing inability to solve their anger, fears, guilt,
their depressed or hopeless feelings about their fate of having to
raise a crippled child. The past histories of these parents often
show that they grew up with a handicapped sibling, such as a
hemophiliac brother, or that they lost another child due to illness
--not infrequently hemophilia. Another reason for becoming a
rejecting parent is serious psychopathology of the parents, including alcoholism and sociopathy. These family constellations
pose those rare instances when the hemophilia care team might have
to suggest at least a temporary placement of the hemophiliac in
a foster home or a residential center.

Finally, we have those families which are characterized by longstanding psychological conflicts between the parents or between the parents and their children, and where the hemophiliac boy serves as a conflict avoidance tool or scapegoat, that is, longstanding family problems get hidden behind the child and his chronic illness. It is rather common to find that a hemophiliac and his concerned mother are allied against the father in a firm coalition. In such instances, the role of the excluded father usually means that he takes very little interest in his son. He has given up trying to influence the raising of his son. There are situations where the spouse dyad is united against the hemophiliac boy. This may be manifested by the parents watching the boy all the time or con- tinually correcting and helping him. In focusing all their attention on their sick, special child, the parents can detour their own conflicts, conflicts which they cannot face and deal with.

When the family functioning is characterized by longstanding maladaptive patterns, ranging from overprotectiveness to rejection and conflict avoidance, family therapy sessions often are fruitful. Here, the therapist will call attention to various dysfunctional family units and coalitions. The therapist might assist the parents in setting up clear guidelines for the emergency home treat- ment of the hemophiliac. The therapist might uncover problems that involve the healthy siblings of the hemophiliac. The overall approach aims at removing the hemophiliac boy as the sole symptom bearer of his family, decreasing his centrality and his power to manipulate the family. The hemophiliac boy should be helped to function as an equal, as responsible for good functioning of his family as his siblings are.

More recent developments in the area of primary prevention of psychosocial problems of families with hemophilia include the female hemophilia carrier's right to abortion and freedom of parenthood; the issue of parents adapting a nonhemophiliac after having borne a hemophiliac son; the prospect of hemophelia home therapy requiring screening of the emotional stability and medical understanding of the family subsystems.

In terms of secondary prevention, we note the situations of serious maladaptation to hemophilia such as risk taking, dare-devil- like attitudes, and passive dependent personality development. These situations usually require psychiatric intervention.

The hemophilia health care team members require continuous education about the various family stress factors that are associated with raising a hemophiliac boy. His family requires ongoing, consistent medical care, and psychosocial support. Robert Louis Stevenson, himself a sufferer from a chronic illness, wrote: "Life is not a matter of holding good cards, but of playing

a poor hand well." With regard to "playing a poor hand well," the
maturation of the child's mind, that is, his cognitive functions,
and the existence of stable family functioning and open communication
are our foremost allies in securing a normal psychosocial development of the hemophiliac.

Summary

Hemophilia is a disease that shares unique problems with
genetic diseases in general, yet shares many more problems with
other chronic diseases. The fear of genetic transmission is a
special stress for parents, as is the possibility of being a
carrier for the female siblings. Similarly, there are special
problems for the hemophiliac child as well as problems shared with
all chornically ill children.

In this paper, three areas were highlighted: First, the way
of using an open rather than a closed systems model to understand
the various interactions operating with childhood hemophilia.
Second, the way of using Piaget's cognitive developmental model
to guide the health professionals in their interactions with and
expectations of the developing child with hemophilia. And, third,
the way of using a model of family dysfunctioning in order to
develop intervention strategies with the relatively small number
of poorly dysfunctioning families with a hemophiliac child. In
all three areas, the problems of the genetically transmitted
disease brings some unique aspects; yet much in these perspectives
is useful and pertinent to the larger group of chronically ill
children. These parameters can enhance the physician's ability to
help the chronically ill children and their families master the ongoing stressful factors associated with the disorders.

REFERENCES

Agle, D. P. and Mattsson, A. Psychological complications of hemo-
    philia. In: M. Hilgartner (Ed.) Progress in Pediatric
    Hematology-Oncology, Vol. 1. Massachusetts: Publishing
    Sciences Group, pp. 137-150, 1976.
Bertalanffy, L. V. General systems theory--a critical review.
    In: W. Buckley (Ed.) Modern Systems Research for the Behavioral
    Scientist. Chicago: Aldine Publishing Company, 1968.
Elkind, D. Children and Adolescents, Second Edition: Interpretive
    Essays on Jean Piaget. New York: Oxford University Press,
    1974.
Erikson, E. H. Identity: Youth and Crisis. Monograph. New York:
    Norton and Company, 1978.
Mattsson, A. Long-term physical illness in childhood: A challenge
    to psychosocial adaptation. Pediatrics, 50:801-811, 1972.

Mattsson, A. Psychophysiologic study of bleeding and adaptation in
    young hemophiliacs. In: E. J. Anthony (Ed.) Explorations in
    Child Psychiatry, New York: Plenum Publishing Corporation,
    pp. 227-246, 1975.
Minuchin, S., Baker, L., Rosman, B. L. A conceptual model of
    psychosomatic illness in children. Archives of General
    Psychiatry, 32:1021-1038, 1975.

"HEMOPHILIAC"--A DEPERSONALIZING TERM: DISCUSSION OF DR. MATTSSON'S
PAPER

Michael B. Rothenberg, M.D.

University of Washington School of Medicine

Seattle, Washington

I feel that Dr. Mattsson's combination of systems theory and
developmental approaches provides us with a marvelously comprehensive
and flexible conceptualization for understanding, preventing or
treating psychosocial problems of the patient and family dealing
with chronic and/or life-threatening illness.

I would like to add that I believe it's critical for us to stay
tuned in to the reactions of the health care providers in these
situations. It seems to me that feelings of frustration, helplessness and hopelessness in health care providers can have a profound
effect on the family's ability to deal with a chronic illness such
as hemophilia. Thus, I would urge us to stay in touch with our
own feelings, as part of the primary prevention of dysfunctional
family and patient responses to chronic illness.

Finally, I must take exception to the use of the word "hemophiliac." For over twenty-five years, I have constantly reminded
myself and urged my colleagues in the health care professions to make
every effort to avoid referring to children by the noun represented
by their illness, i.e., "diabetic," "asthmatic," "leukemic," etc.
It seems to me that even those of us from the behavioral sciences
run the risk of being subtly drawn into depersonalizing our patients
to some extent when we begin to refer to them as "cystics" or "hemophiliacs" or whatever the case may be. Certainly, our colleagues
in the health care professions who are less aware of such self-
protective mechanisms do indeed use the noun representing the name
of the disease in a manner that clearly depersonalizes and even
dehumanizes patients. We are dealing with <u>children</u> who have these
dreadful illnesses, and if we are successfully to meet their develop-

157

mental and psychosocial needs and those of their families, we must let ourselves feel the impact of what this means from the most profoundly human point of view.

IDENTITY AND THE LABEL OF HEMOPHILIAC: GENERAL DISCUSSION

Dr. Mattsson

I want to thank Dr. Rothenberg for his remarks. I agree very
much with his comments about the use of the word hemophilia. At
the National Hemophiliac Foundation, parents regularly bring up
the matter, but feel it is relatively unimportant. In part, perhaps,
they feel this because medical people are bent on using these terms.
It's the same with the diagnostic terms in mental illness.

Dr. Christ

There is little argument about the need for nonpejorative
labels. I'm wondering about the identity of the youngsters: To
what extent do they incorporate the term and the state hemophilia
in their identity? I would suspect that the life-long and hereditary
aspect would enhance the acceptance of hemophilia as a part of their
basic identity rather than as an intrusion, as, for example, a
youngster with a broken leg might feel. I have never, for example,
encountered a child who developed even a transient identity as a
broken leg or as a leukemic.

Dr. Mattsson

Children are constantly referred to as the leukemic or the
compound tibial fracture by medical staff.

Dr. Christ

That's true.

Dr. Berlin

As the broken leg in bed four. Absolutely.

Dr. Christ

I wonder if there is one continuum in developing an identity
that incorporates a disease, from the most unlikely, like a transient

159

acute illness or a broken leg, through a chronic one like leukemia
or cerebral palsy, to one that is both chronic and hereditary, like
sickle cell anemia or hemophilia? Embedded in this question is the
other one: is it more or less adaptive to accept or develop an
identity that incorporates a chronic illness such as sickle cell
disease or hemophilia?

Nancy Salander: Audience Member--Social Worker

One of the concerns that the parents as well as the young men
with hemophilia express is: If they lose this identity, they lose
the sense of advocacy and, in essence, society's willingness to
provide funds. This is a real issue among them, because in Rhode
Island, we have legislation that provides funds for their care. On
the other hand, another concern that some of us shared last week,
who were together with staffs of other hemophilia centers, was the
creation of a sense of entitlement and uniqueness that, in the long
run, may well boomerang. It is making treatment very difficult,
because they are holding on to this sense of uniqueness. They resist
more or less getting into the mainstream. I wish one of you could
comment on this.

Dr. Rothenberg

This is precisely the point that I am making. I thank you for
really extending it because I just limited my comment in the critique
of Dr. Mattsson's paper to the issue of depersonalization and de-
humanization. You brought up what I think is, perhaps, even more
important--the degree to which this identification of oneself or
one's children with the disease can interfere with the integration,
not only of the child, but of the family into the mainstream of
society. It can lead to severe isolation.

Nancy Salander: Audience Member--Social Worker

We are definitely finding some young men and their families
unwilling to give up this uniqueness and this label. It's their
cause for being--for existence.

Dr. Mattsson

I have had the opportunity of working with the National Hemophilia Foundation, the Diabetes Association, and the Cystic Fibrosis
Organization. When you meet with their members, you see examples
of what you are describing. However, I also meet successful
adaptors, be they physicians, artists, businessnen, who say "I am
diabetic", "I am a hemophiliac", and so on. There is no easy
one-to-one relationship between identifying as a diabetic, and doing
poorly or doing well.

Dr. Christ

    I suspect that the prognosis of a chronic disease affects the
incorporation of it in one's identity formation, as well as
whether we would perceive such an identity to be adaptive or
maladaptive. Given the dramatic change in the prognosis of hemophilia in the past ten years, is there any information that throws
light on the importance of prognosis in the "healthy" acceptance of
an identity including the disease? Specifically, has there been a
change in the way the identity of oneself "with hemophilia" or as
a "hemophiliac" develops as a result of the improved prognosis?

Dr. Mattsson

    Parents and young patients talk about the tremendous relief
they experienced when the new plasma fractions became available.
Also, when home care became possible, there were gains in being
able to work, in being able to go to school without interruptions,
gains in self control, in self management, and in family cohesive-
ness. There are several studies going on in the country comparing
families of young hemophiliacs on home care and not on home care,
which try to tease out some of the things Dr. Christ is mentioning.

    Because they are on home care, these patients are not as
connected with the centers. Consequently, they develop a sense
almost of "I really don't have hemophilia." As a consequence, in
some instances they are not taking as good care of themselves as
they should. Also there is still the very real danger and fear
of cerebral hemorrhage.

Dr. Hal Strolick: Audience Member--Family Physician

    What role do you see families and organizations such as
National Hemophilia Foundation having in primary and secondary
prevention regarding self-help, self-caring, and the families
helping each other?

Dr. Mattsson

    I appreciate a question like this one. I have been very
fortunate in being able to help young families and not so young
families with hemophilia to organize themselves into self-help
groups. Experienced parents may act as "lay counselors" on the
phone and in the office with young families during the first couple
of months after their son has been diagnosed. They can be very
helpful with regard to practical issues of raising a hemophiliac
boy. These parents can acknowledge with the inexperienced parents
that they have been through the same situations and feelings. Sometimes, however, we have seen that boomerang. I'll never forget

a young family of a two year old hemophiliac boy joining an established group of six other families of hemophiliacs. Not only had
they been meeting for a couple of months, but their sons were all
over four to five years old. They greeted that young family by
telling them horror stories of all kinds of medical problems they
had to look forward to. You have to be very careful when you select
families with the same illness as helpers, and warn them about
these potential problems. Associations such as the National
Hemophilia Foundation, with many chapters throughout the country,
have done a fantastic amount of good work. Thanks to the present
organizations, some twenty states have passed legislation, with
each of these states providing between two and three hundred
thousand dollars for the care of hemophiliacs.

Nancy Salander: Audience Member--Social Worker

    That's why they don't want to give up the term hemophiliac.

Dr. Rothenberg

    Yes, but I think that's a break in logic. You don't have
to have the term hemophiliac to have an effective group. I would
just like to emphasize what Dr. Mattsson just said: I have experience
both with the National Sudden Infant Death Group and the Candlelight
Group. The latter is exclusively devoted to children with various
forms of cancer. There is always the danger that the group, simply
due to a lack of education about more sophisticated psychosocial
and psychodynamic issues, can inadvertently do damage to its own
members. That's why I try to achieve a balance in the group. I
feel it is essential that the parents and other lay people in these
groups intelligently use medical consultation. Historically, there
has been a battle with physicians feeling in charge of some of these
diseases, hence very reluctant for parents to get involved at all.
On the other hand, it's equally dangerous to let the parents totally
loose, and not use good counsel about what to do with a new set of
young parents who get dropped into an ongoing group like the one
described by Dr. Mattsson.

THE EFFECT OF A CHILD'S CHRONIC ILLNESS ON THE FAMILY

Michael B. Rothenberg, M. D.*

University of Washington School of Medicine

Seattle, Washington

Chronic illness in children may cause a disturbance in what may be called the "psychosocial metabolism" of the entire family. The baseline, homeostatic state of the family's psychosocial metabolism will often be shifted by the child's chronic illness. This conceptualization can be examined in two major areas: (a) The affective issues for the child and his family, and (b) The socio-economic and physical environmental issues for the entire family.

Affective Issues for the Child and His Family

FAGS is a mnemonic device focusing on four reactions of children to illness and/or hospitalization. These reactions--fear, anger, guilt, and sadness--occur to some extent every time a child becomes ill and are most prominent in relation to serious illness or hospitalization. The FAGS syndrome is shared by the child, his family, and the health professional. The syndrome can affect everyone's response to the child's illness and even the course of the illness itself.

When a child becomes ill, either acutely or chronically, the entire family experiences a greater or lesser amount of fear. This is occurring particularly today in relation to the fragmented and stressful society in which we are all living. These fears apply to

_____

*The author acknowledges with gratitude the editorial assistance of Ms Jo Lamport in the preparation of this chapter from transcribed material.

163

a number of different issues. The initial fear about what is wrong
can often be resolved. The family then has fears about what is going
to be done for the child and whether in fact anything will be able
to be done. The parents and caretakers of the child may fear that
they have failed somehow in their caretaking role and that this
failure has led to the child becoming ill. Caretakers may also fear
the disapproval of the health care provider for allowing the child
to become ill. Parents and caretakers may fear that they will somehow prove to be inadequate or unsuccessful in dealing with the
challenge of the child's illness or hospitalization. It is not
just the family that is experiencing these fears, but obviously
also the patient himself and often the health care providers as well.

It is often very difficult to recognize and subsequently
accept the degree of anger associated with the child's illness.
Anger is generated towards oneself, as the caretaker, for somehow
allowing this child to become ill. The family may show anger at
"the system" for all of its multifaceted impingements on the family.
This begins to interrelate with socio-economic and physical environmental issues. Anger is often directed at health care providers
who are not available enough, responsive enough, or knowledgeable
enough to deal rapidly enough with the many aspects of the child's
illness. Most difficult of all, in situations where the child is
chronically ill, and especially in cases of chronic life-threatening
illnesses, anger is generated by the family towards the child patient
himself. For example, when a child has an illness which everybody
knows will be fatal, it is rare for the family, caretakers, and even
health care providers, to avoid feeling irritation and anger towards
this child who will neither get well nor get the illness over with
and die, in spite of all the effort and experience of difficulty
that has been manifested on the child's behalf.

In our society, guilt and anger have become strongly linked.
When one gets angry at a child who is ill, one is likely to feel
guilty as well, and this particular guilt is quite unpleasant. The
source of this pain, the unpleasant emotion of guilt, is the very
child at whom one just got angry, and this makes one angry at the
child all over again. This vicious circle of anger and guilt begins
to flow rather smoothly and tends to escalate very rapidly in its
intensity. Family groups, siblings, parents, caretakers, grandparents, and others, significant and otherwise, get caught in this
kind of vicious circle. •They often feel so distressed about this,
and so convinced that there must be something wrong with them to
even experience such feelings in relation to a seriously ill child,
that they cannot share these feelings with anybody else in their
environment and therefore are unable to get any support. It is not
unusual to discover a family where several members are experiencing
the same agony of anger and guilt and each is convinced that he or
she is the only one having such an experience. Progressive isolation

from other family members results for fear of having these feelings discovered.

Sadness is a reaction to loss. The family experiences a loss of the child (due to his hospitalization) and of normal routines. It is often difficult to distinguish between sadness and depression. Although depression may involve loss, its distinguishing characteristics is that it always involves withheld anger and therefore demands a different therapeusis.

Families who have become depressed around a child's chronic illness can be successfully helped if they are able to ventilate their angry feelings and discharge them at whomever they are directed, including health care providers. Every child and family member has some basic questions that may have contributed to this depression and that need to be answered in the course of the child's illness. The following questions are always present but seldom explicitly stated:

1. What does the child have?
2. How did he get it?
3. Why did he get it?
4. What will be done about it?
5. When will the child get well and come home?

The first two questions can usually be answered through basic explanation to the parents and through them, siblings and extended family groups. The third question differs significantly from the second because it begins to include the issues of fear and guilt. The fourth question includes the whole welter of diagnostic and therapeutic procedures which are about to begin and may continue especially in cases of chronic illness, for an indefinite length of time. The fifth question, "When will the child get well?" or "When will the child come home?" is often the only question explicitly stated by either parents or sick children. Its repetition signifies a good deal of anxiety and the probable inability of the patient or family to articulate the other questions.

Clinical interaction in identifying and answering these questions is necessary to help families understand the affective issues of their child's illness. The third person approach is often very helpful, e.g. "Many times familes in your situation find themselves wondering about how their child got this illness, or what role did his sibling play in the incident that preceded the onset of this illness?" This allows the family, and again through them, the siblings and extended family group, to understand the affective issues surrounding the patient's illness, to begin to share and ventilate their feelings, and to mediate, to some extent, the impact of the child's chronic illness on the family's psychosocial metabolism.

It is important to keep in mind that adults, as well as children, are involved in four major areas of growth and development at any given time. These four areas are: physical, intellectual, emotional, and social. The impact of a child's chronic illness on a family will often be heavily determined by where each family member is in terms of his or her own developmental milestones or particular developmental crises at the time the child's illness is discovered, and often later as the illness progresses through remissions or relapses. A systematic approach to the psychosocial growth and development of both children and their families can provide a sound theoretical basis for clinical comprehensive care.

Socioeconomic and Physical Environmental Issues

Many pediatricians have not been trained to assess or respond to the socioeconomic and physical environmental issues which confront the family of a seriously or chronically ill child. Most of these issues have yet to be examined in an organized fashion, perhaps because they can appear to be very obvious and require only common sense responses on a superficial level. However, they often have a much deeper impact on the child, and the family, in the course of the illness.

Chronic illness effects a chronic financial strain on most families in this country today. Families who are neither very poor nor very rich must mortgage their entire holdings before the scale of the bills for the child's care begins to change.

Chronic illness also places severe demands for physical labor on parents and other caretakers. In families where the seriously ill child is being cared for in the home, physical labor is assumed by one or two individuals at best, 24 hours a day, seven days a week. Incredible stress is produced by the subsequent chronic physical fatigue. When the child is hospitalized, physical labor and care are divided among rotating shifts of hospital personnel but parents and caretakers are nevertheless often literally being worn out by simply being there, being awake too much of the time, and helping wherever they can.

Major geographical moves are often precipitated by the necessity of bringing a chronically ill child closer to a medical center. For most families, such a move constitutes a major stress. Physical dislocation frequently occurs within a household. When the seriously ill child must have special sleeping or care quarters, the rest of the family must rearrange their own sleeping spaces, and often schedules, to accommodate the child. For example, a child requiring home kidney dialysis will need a bedroom on the first floor with special plumbing installations to support the dialysis equipment.

I would like to make special mention of some of the early research efforts that are being made in this country to develop more hard data about the impact of a child's chronic illness on the family. Stein and Reissman (1980) at Albert Einstein College of Medicine in New York have been attempting to develop objective measures of the impact on a family of a child's chronic illness. They have been able to identify, quite specifically, clusters of responses in whole groups of families that fall out in terms of familial responses, personal responses, financial responses, emotional responses, etc. I would emphasize that this is work in progress, but the early data does provide objective verification of what has been clinically believed for many years.

Interview with a Chronically Ill Child and His Parents

The following transcript contains approximately twenty minutes edited out of a one-hour videotaped interview. This interview was conducted as part of a weekly comprehensive care case conference at our hospital, for the pediatric house staff as well as for others who would like to attend. The child and, whenever possible, the child's family are interviewed live, in front of the group, with a three-fold purpose; to demonstrate: (a) comprehensive care interviewing techniques from a pediatric point of view; (b) normal and pathological growth and development issues; and (c) approaches to dispositional decision-making about such children and their families from a comprehensive care point of view.

It should be noted that we define comprehensive care as the systematic inclusion of psychosocial dynamics and personality development in the practice of pediatrics, in a family and community context.

All names, other than mine, have been changed to maintain privileged communications.

Dr. Rothenberg: Hi Stan, I am Dr. Rothenberg.

Stan: Hello.

Dr. R.:   How do you do?

Stan: Fine.

Dr. R.:   Thank you very much for coming to talk to me.

Stan: You are welcome. (Stan gives hug to Dr. R.)

Dr. R.:   Okay, thank you. You are pretty good. Hi,
                   who is that guy? Do you remember him? This one
                   here? This man right here, you remember?

Stan:	No.
Dr. R.:	Dr. Barnes, Dr. Ed Barnes, that's who he is.
Dr. B.:	Do I get a hug too?
Stan:	Yes, you get a hug too.
Dr. R.:	Oh boy, you are strong today aren't you?
Stan:	Yes.
Dr. R.:	Stan? Excuse me, I want you to tell me who this man is right here.
Stan:	I want to sit beside you.
Dr. R.:	Remember his name? Hm?
Stan:	I want to sit beside you. Ah, ah.
Dr. R.:	Dr. Gold
Stan:	Dr. Gold.
Dr. R.:	Yep. Stan, could I read those? You got two signs on you and I haven't even read them. Can I read your signs? (I just want to tell you this is a 9 year old boy who has had a brain tumor operated on.) Okay, that says Stan and it gives your address and your phone number. And this one says in case of medical emergency, call Dr. Kent.
Stan:	Miss is my dog.
Dr. R.:	What's that?
Stan:	This is my dog.
Dr. R.:	Your dog? This is my dog?
Stan:	No, this is my dog.
Dr. R.:	I don't understand what you are saying--Misses? Miss is your dog? Now I understand.
Stan:	Hm, Hm.
Dr. R.:	How long have you had your dog?

Stan:	I don't know.
Dr. R.:	A long time?
Stan:	Maybe, maybe not.
Dr. R.:	What kind of dog is Miss? Special kind?
Stan:	No, Miss is a big dog.
Dr. R.:	She is a big dog. What color is she?
Stan:	I don't know.
Dr. R.:	Think about it for a minute.
Stan:	I don't want to.
Dr. R.:	All right. What color is your sweater?
Stan:	I don't know.
Dr. R.:	You don't know what color that is?
Stan:	Uh, uh.
Dr. R.:	I have a feeling that you do and you are teasing me. No?
Stan:	I can do patty-cake.
Dr. R.:	You can?
Stan:	Yes.
Dr. R.:	You want to do it?
Stan:	Watch me do patty-cake.
Dr. R.:	I'll watch you.
Stan:	Patty-cake, patty-cake, baker's man, bake me a cake as fast as you can, roll it and prick it with a B for Baby and me.
Dr. R.:	That's very good!

(Note: Stan leaves and parents enter room.)

Dr. R.:   We have had from Dr. Barnes and Dr. Gold a brief
               sort of bird's eye summary of what's happened to
               Stan since he was three. And maybe a good place
               to start, though I don't want you to feel that
               you have to be limited to there at all, is with
               a question, and apparently it is a question, about
               what kinds of changes you folks have been noticing
               more recently or most recently?

Mother: You mean in Stan himself?

Dr. R.:   In Stan. You see the impression I get is that there
               are some interests that he has shown in the past
               that he no longer has. Question mark as to whether
               there are some skills that he has had that he's
               lost or lost part of. And that there's more
               question mark about.

Mother: Skills--he was never old enough to accomplish any.
               He does what he was able to do mostly when he was
               three. But after that, no. No skills.

Father: No, he hasn't acquired any new skills.

Mother: He could draw, but he doesn't do that anymore.
               He scribbles. When he was three, before he was ill,
               he could draw very well.

Dr. R.:   Before he was ill?

Mother: He could make stick men which would be normal at
               that time. No more.

Father: There was a period of time since he became sick
               that he has drawn these little stick men, but
               that's been quite a while since he has done that
               now, even.

Mother: He really knows no, I would say no skills at all.

Dr. R.:   Dr. Barnes mentioned that I think it was you
               Mrs. W who had made the statement that it seems
               that we lose a little bit of him each time he
               has surgery. I don't know if that's a correct
               paraphrase.

Mother: Yes, that's our way of putting it. It seems that
               there is one more thing in his body that no longer
               functions. Or his mind is a little bit more gone
               or he is just not the same boy any longer. We've

noticed that he may come in more quiet and less communicative.

Dr. R.:   Wheelchair? Do you use a wheelchair?

Mother: We take him in a wheelchair when we go like to the fair or to the zoo because he tires so easily and we walk a half a block and then he really is ready to quit.

Dr. R.:   I see.

Mother: It's easier to just put him in a wheelchair and take him that way.

Dr. R.:   I understand that in fact sort of the whole family, your other three children, along with the two of you, have all pitched in over the years in sharing at least some of the babysitting and at least sharing in chores with you.

Father: The babysitting--to just hire a "babysitter" is almost out of the question. Number one, a lot of parents (i.e. of babysitters) don't want their young children, their teenage children (i.e. babysitters) to have the responsibility that Stan's care might bring out.

Mother: He could have a seizure or something like that. It would frighten them.

Father: Right, and it wouldn't be fair to ask them to. Our children have grown up with it. At least the girl and the younger of the two other boys.

Mother: The 15 year old boy, he is very good with him.

Father: They know the set procedure they would have to go through. And the other alternative to a babysitter is to hire a practical or registered nurse, which would obviously become impossible in terms of economics.

Dr. R.:   Sure. What about the kids, the other kids, in terms of their relationship and their feelings about Stan? How would you describe that?

Mother: Well, with our oldest boy, it is a little bit difficult for him. Stan was his favorite when he was a baby and after he got sick, he has never

really been able to accept the way Stan is now.
It bothers him. But the other two, I think maybe
they love him a bit more.

Dr. R.:   And the oldest one? Let's see, he would have been
               at least 16 when Stan became ill.

Mother: He was 16 when Stan was born.

Dr. R.:   So 19 when Stan was ill, which meant he was just
               getting out of high school.

Mother: He has been away. He wasn't even living home at
               that time. He was working away from home and he
               hasn't really lived at home since. It is just
               recently that he moved back home again so he hasn't
               been around him a lot, these past few years.

Dr. R.:   What led to his being out of the home and working?

Mother: He went on a summer job and from there he went
               to college and then in the service and he was
               married and now he is getting a divorce and is
               back home again.

Dr. R.:   I see.

Father: He wasn't around in any continuity during the time
               that Stan became sick.

Mother: None of the times when he was ill at all.

Father: And I think partly it's just that he hasn't found
               a way of accepting the fact that Stan is not the
               same little boy that he was when he left.

Dr. R.:   In contrast to this then, the other two kids really
               seem to be able to work with him and feel more
               comfortable. Have they had any problems, as is
               often seen in families with a chronically ill
               child? Have the other kids had any problems in
               terms of bringing other kids home for dates or for
               parties or whatever?

Mother: None whatsoever.

Father: We, in fact, have felt very fortunate. I guess
               you might say our daughter is a little bit of an
               introvert so she has not had a "social life" more

or less by her own choice, a lot of it. The other little guy--all of his friends have really been very tolerant in accepting Stan's problems.

Dr. R.:   Are you religious people?

Mother: Well, we believe, I mean we don't constantly go to Church, but we believe, yes.

Dr. R.:   I ask that because when you raised the question, "Why?", that often people will find themselves asking God why, if they believe.

Mother: Well, I guess that's what I meant. But I didn't do that very long.

Father: That was at the time of our first knowing that there was not going to be a positive, a medical cure for Stan's problem.

Dr. R.:   When was that, by the way?

Mother: They told us then, that it was inoperable and that he would continue to have problems.

Dr. R.:   This was after the surgery?

Mother: After the second surgery. He told us then that he couldn't remove it and that we would have continued problems. I've gotten so that I can anticipate, in fact I've tried to outguess the doctors sometimes when he's really sick, and I usually come out right, which is a bad thing to do, but I do it anyway.

Dr. R.:   Why is it bad?

Mother: I don't know. They say it is not good to have a little bit of knowledge about something like that, but I do it anyway. I can't help it.

Father: I guess maybe one of the things we have had a little difficulty in communicating, not particularly to Dr. Kent because he is very concise in his explanations, very understanding, but to some of the doctors that we have encountered, we have had a little problem getting it across to them that we do know a little of Stan's problems and if there is something going on we want to know about it. We don't want to be kept in the dark. We would

like a minute-by-minute resume as it were. Even
if it's bad news, we want to know.

Mother: I just go wild if I know something is going on and
              I don't know what's happening.

Dr. R.:   I am going to ask you a tough one. In looking
              back over the past six years, what would you, and
              I want each of you to answer this separately if
              you would, what would each of you see as the
              toughest single problem you had to deal with
              through this whole thing? What aspect of all of
              this has been the hardest one for each of you?

Mother: For me, it's when he goes to surgery, I think.

Dr. R.:   What's particularly tough about that?

Mother: Just knowing that anything could happen, and he
              probably wouldn't make it through.

Dr. R.:   So, specifically that he may die during a
              surgical. Mr. W, what's been the toughest aspect
              for you as you look back over the years?

Father: Well, I share the fears of course at any given
              surgery time. I think the toughest thing for me
              is knowing that Momma here has to live with this
              24 hours a day as it were, and I feel a little
              helpless, in fact, I feel a lot helpless about that.
              I can go to work. I have to go to work, and I've
              reached the point where I can immerse myself in
              my work enough, that at least for that period of
              the day, I am free of the hourly worry and that's
              the toughest thing for me to live with, is knowing
              that I can't do anything to help, really.

Dr. R.:   I understand that one of the things that has been
              upsetting to both of you is that on at least a
              couple of occasions, you've had the sense of, if
              not out and out pressure being put on you, at
              least having to deal with the recommendations of
              physicians to institutionalize Stan, and that this
              has been very, very difficult.

Mother: Been very for me.

Dr. R.:   I wonder if we could talk a little about that, in
              terms of how you both felt, if you can kind of look
              back on it when this was first laid on you, if

you will.

Mother: I was very unhappy with the doctor to even suggest
            it.

Dr. R.:   It came as quite a shock?

Father: Yes, nothing we had ever contemplated you know.
            And it made...it seemed as if our efforts in doing
            for Stan and in keeping him and securing medical
            care for him and everything were sort of pointless.
            You know, if they are going to, if someone is going
            to say, well okay this we've done as far as we can
            and now we think an institution should handle the
            problem, what have we been struggling for, for
            these last six years? My personal feeling is
            there's too many people in this world are willing
            to let institutions handle what are specifically
            their problems and it just didn't set well at all.

Dr. R.:   In essence, you know, I get the very real sense
            that while certainly it's not something that is the
            foremost thing in your thinking every day of your
            lives, and it couldn't be, nevertheless in the
            background, you've been living for some time
            with the...

Mother: Time bomb.

Dr. R.:   That's right, you use that expression. As a
            matter of fact, I've made a little note of that
            'cause Dr. Barnes mentioned that too. What I
            specifically wanted to say though was the time
            bomb, if I hear it right, is the issue of death,
            whether it's sudden, unexpected through some
            hemorrhage because the tumor invades an artery or
            infringes on...

Mother: No, it's attached to the artery and we know some-
            thing could happen there and that was explained to
            us.

Father: The reason that it was inoperable as I understand
            it was its involvement with...they mentioned the
            name of the artery and I can't remember it now.

Mother: Me neither.

Dr. R.:   If it's an artery, that's what counts, because that
            means trouble. To what extent are the other kids

aware of this issue? That is, that in a sense
you're dealing with the issue of death and dying
really every day of the collective family's life?

Mother: They realize that if Stan gets sick, it's possible
               that this could happen to him, but we don't live
               with it. I mean we live with it but we don't just
               sit down and talk about it. I mean they just know.

Father: They have been told that Stan is not ever going
               to be any better and the younger boy, the little
               guy, he is quite sensitive, he is a little more
               prone to show things than the others and he worries
               a lot. He is a worry wart by nature anyway. Always
               was. His school work would fall off.

Mother: But he is fully aware of it. We could lose him.
               I think Fred will have more of a problem when we
               lose Stan than he will have now.

Dr. R.:   Does he actually share a room with Stan for
               example?

Mother: No, Stan sleeps in our room. We've been thinking
               of moving him in, but now he is seizuring a lot
               again so we have kept him in our room in a crib.
               For sometimes he will get up and wander.

Father: We live in an open split-level type place. He
               could, you know, if he were up wandering around,
               we would want to know about it.

Dr. R.:   Has that been a problem just in terms of your own
               sleep patterns?

Mother: Not recently. Well, during the seizuring, there
               for a long time, he was having quite a problem
               sleeping and he was sleeping only about two hours
               out of every 24, but then we slept in shifts
               around the house then. I would stay up all night
               with him, and then all day, and then somebody
               when they, when my daughter came home from school,
               then she would take over so that I could go to bed
               and then Daddy would come home and have dinner and
               then when he came to bed, I would get back up
               again. So we really worked it out very well.

Dr. R.:   Boy, how long did that go on?

Mother: Oh, that went on for about six months.

Father: I was going to say closer to a year.

Mother: Then I guess maybe so.

                 (Dr. R. refers to the fact that family moved a great
                 distance away from a rural area to a medical center
                 where Stan could get his care.)

Dr. R.:   Was that move a problem for you?

Mother: It didn't bother me. I don't know if it
                 bothered him (i.e. Father).

Father: It bothered me because I am not really a city
                 boy and it meant coming back to the city.

Mother: I am just so grateful to have the care for Stan
                 that is available to us here.

Father: Personally, starting over again, just aside from
                 or outside the problems of Stan's care, starting
                 over again.

Mother: Economically, it was difficult.

Father: Economically, I think that it will always scare
                 a man.

Dr. R.:   Often parents express to us this feeling, "I must
                 confess to you doctor that for my child's sake,
                 I find myself wishing it were over at times."

Mother: Yes, I do.

Father: The only rationalization we can apply, and it's
                 not an answer, is the fact that Stan doesn't know
                 that anything's wrong.

Mother: He is totally unaware that anything is wrong.

Father: He does not realize he is sick. He has his own
                 little world and he thinks that in his little
                 world that this is the way things are.

Mother: I know he does. I mean he's got a problem. I know
                 he does suffer even though he may be unaware of
                 it and it's hard for us, as parents, to just stand
                 aside and see this.

DISCUSSION

Stan's illness had more than a little to do with the growth and
development of each of his siblings. In fact, the older brother of
the patient did not sequentially leave home, go to work, and go to
college as presented by the mother. He left home to go to college
and he was working in order to stay in college. He had to work
increasingly longer hours when there wasn't enough money from
home to keep him in college because Stan's illness was draining so
much of the family's money. The boy then dropped out of college,
had a terrible row with the family, joined the Army, etc.

The parents chose to see their daughter being "naturally introverted" as having nothing whatsoever to do with her brother's
condition. They also chose to see the younger boy as being a
naturally sensitive, caretaking person who would have assumed the
role he assumed, in terms of caretaking for Stan, in any case.

Stan's parents also experienced personal difficulties. When
Stan was first diagnosed, he was brought from Idaho to Seattle
and had his first surgery, which he survived. The family was told
that there was a tumor that could not be entirely removed because
it was involved with one of the arteries. At this point, the father
left the family, was separated from them for a period of several
months, and then returned, primarily because of his intense sense
of personal responsibility. This is demonstrated in the interview
in his brief comment about society in general, and his belief that
folks are too willing to let institutions take over what should be
their own individual responsibility.

The effect of the sleeping arrangements on the marital relationship was profound. There was in fact no sex life between these
parents and there had been none for some three years prior to
this interview. It was not clear how much of this was the direct
result of the caretaking necessities in accommodating Stan's
sleeping patterns and how much of it had to do with the couple's
ongoing relationship.

The family had certainly been far more impinged upon in its
total growth and development by Stan's illness than might be evident
in this edited segment of the interview. This did not, however,
prevent them from showing enormous strength through the very end.
They kept Stan at home, in a slowly deteriorating state, as long
as they possibly could, at which time they brought him to the
hospital where he died three days later.

REFERENCES

Stein, R.E.K. and Riessman, C.K. The Development of an Impact-on-
     Family Scale: Preliminary Findings. Medical Care 18 (4),
     pp. 465-472, 1980.

YEARS OF CHALLENGE: A FAMILY LIVES WITH CHRONIC ILLNESS: DISCUSSION

OF DR. ROTHENBERG'S PAPER

John Sargent, M. D.

Philadelphia Child Guidance Clinic

Philadelphia, Pennsylvania

It has been a homily in medicine that we must learn from our patients. It is rare, though, that we have an opportunity as excellent as that which Dr. Rothenberg and the family he interviews offer us today. I would first like to comment on Dr. Rothenberg's approach to the parents and their son. He is warm, friendly and direct with the family. His respectful questioning permits them to describe openly and poignantly their experience over the previous six years and to relate directly the difficulties they have lived through and continue to face. I would also like to stress that Dr. Rothenberg is an informed interviewer. He brings an appreciation of the potential effects of an illness of this magnitude on an entire family to the interview. He then amplifies this knowledge immensely by gathering and organizing information from this family's physicians. This prior understanding enables him to present, through the interview, the challenges, disappointments and triumphs of their lives. I would strongly encourage those who would support families through similar experiences to emulate Dr. Rothenberg's depth of understanding of the home environment of the chronically ill child and his warm, respectful manner in meeting with them.

Every family with an ill child is presented with both the general challenges of chronic illness and long term medical care as well as those that are disease specific. It is especially relevant that Dr. Rothenberg has included in his videotape presentation a brief picture of the affected child. This is clearly a special boy. He is not simply a mentally retarded child. His memory is poor, his articulation often indistinct, his statements are disconnected from those of the interviewer. An understressed challenge of chronic illness for a family is the need to learn directly from the child what he can and cannot do. One cannot rely

179

on either normal expectations of child development nor upon so-called
expert determinations in responding to such individualized skills
and deficiencies. That this family has met this challenge successfully is apparent from the boy's friendly approach to the interviewer, his physical warmth, his well-cared for appearance and his
pleasure in demonstrating a game he enjoys and knows well. It is
only through this knowledge of their child's abilities that a family
can provide the appropriate measure of support and external structure
to encourage development to the child's potential.

This family also relates many other demands which their son's
illness has made upon them. Acute medical emergencies such as
seizures and neurosurgery with its intra- and post-operative dangers
are routinely disruptive for them. Meanwhile, the family lives with
his slow, inexorable loss of skills and the knowledge that the illness will be terminal, with their son's death the predicted outcome
of their efforts.

Dr. Rothenberg rightly inquires about the effects of this
child's illness on his siblings. I do wonder about the daughter
who is "fortunately" introverted and the older brother who has
recently moved home following a divorce and is so affected by his
brother's illness. The listener begins to appreciate the delicate
task of parents to care for a special child, enlist his siblings'
assistance while encouraging their full development and growth,
expecting that they will leave home and live on their own.

The parents report the necessity of observing their son through
the night, having their child sleep in their bedroom regularly.
This kind of sleeping arrangement can easily interrupt or make
difficult normal sexual relations for the parents. This strain,
together with usual requirements that the father continue work,
perhaps even increasing work time to cover added medical expenses,
while the mother attends their child's medical appointments, com-
pounds the demands on the parents. The medical care system,
especially the child's physician, must be aware of these added
stresses and should regularly inquire of both parents how their
marriage and their own lives are faring through the course of the
child's illness. If there are difficulties that are too overwhelming for the parents, additional support and therapy may be
necessary.

This family also states clearly something exceedingly important
for us. This boy is their child and they expect recognition of
that fact from professionals they deal with. They "don't want to
be kept in the dark." At every point through the course of their
son's illness and treatment, they need to know. They want neither
pity nor protectiveness from us. With appropriate information (which
includes reminders of their need to care for themselves also),

they will decide how to balance the priorities of their lives.
Their decisions may seem unusual to us, but it is those decisions
and their actions which provides their efforts with meaning and
rewards.

I am particularly impressed with the mutual support and flexibility of this family. Both husband and wife are involved in the
interview. They answer in concert and the husband clearly respects
and supports his wife's caretaking efforts with their son. One
further feature of this family's experience is the effect of this
child's persistent immaturity upon the developmental process of the
whole family. This is a family with older parents, adolescent
children, yet also requiring significant involvement between the
mother and her ill son, more appropriate for families with young
children. This brings me to my major concern about this family:
What will this mother do when her son does die, as she suddenly
becomes unemployed? Not only will she need support with her grieving, she will need assistance in reorganizing her life. This transition may be difficult for this family. It is a final, little
appreciated challenge of chronic illness.

I have spoken throughout these comments of challenges and
demands for families rather than effects upon families. I consider
this to be an extremely important distinction. Thanks to the efforts
of Dr. Rothenberg and others, we are developing a coherent
appreciation of what families experience with chronically ill children. A further question which must be answered is, "How is this
accomplished?" Different families respond to the same demands in
different ways with different functional results for the family as
a whole and for its individual members. It is through the process
of family interaction that these challenges, which Dr. Rothenberg
has spoken about and demonstrated, are met. It is also through
enhancing or altering family interactions that we can influence the
effects that meeting these demands have upon families.

EXTENDED FAMILY: A VALUABLE SUPPORT : GENERAL DISCUSSION

Dr. Mattsson

I have a couple of questions regarding the parents' last
comments: Both mother and father said that it is difficult for them
to live with the fact that the son himself doesn't seem to know or
comprehend that he is sick. That is fascinating. I wonder what
you did with it or what you thought you might have done with it
over a period of time? Obviously, the parents are approaching the
situation in a number of ways: As parents, they don't know what is
really going to happen to him. None of us knows what is going to
happen to us when we die. We don't want to think the child knows
how ill he is and what is going to happen to him. He doesn't give
us any indication about being aware that he is slowly going downhill.
We are really grateful to him that he does not seem to show that
awareness. All of us who work with children like this one, know
how strikingly successful some of these slowly dying youngsters are
in protecting the whole family from really facing the fact that they
are going to die.

Dr. Christ

An important distinction, however, is what factors are operating
when we, as parents or physicians, "protect" ourselves by not
understanding the child. The probability of our not understanding
the child increases as the child's cognitive level of development is
preoperational, rather than concrete or formal operational, especially if there are additional cognitive difficulties secondary to brain
damage as in this particular youngster.

Dr. Rothenberg

I agree. Dr. Mattsson is making a terribly important point
which is magnificantly illustrated in Myra Langer's The Private
Worlds of Dying Children. This is a beautiful document about dying
children and the extraordinary degree to which the children protect
their parents and their health care providers from the child's own
knowledge that he is in fact dying. In the case I presented, this
little boy was profoundly retarded as a result of his multiple

surgeries and he was functioning at a preoperational level, unable
to deal with the concept of death, certainly, as an irreversible
biological phenomenon.

In the interview I was trying to check out his developmental
level in questioning him about the color of his sweater and having
him count the buttons on his sweater. Clearly, he didn't know
primary colors and he couldn't count. He does as well as he does
because his mother puts in endless hours teaching him such things
as patty-cake. He would keep forgetting it, and then she would
teach it to him again. I am sure that in preparation for this interview, which the parents knew about some time in advance, that he
was tutored for his appearance, and that his mom, with all good
intentions, would have rehearsed all of the few little skills that
he still maintained.

Dr. Dorothy Ramsey: Audience Member

In terms of the physical labor and exhaustion of the family,
have you ever considered a respite approach, where the child is
admitted to an acute care setting for a short period of time to give
the family a break? Would this family accept this kind of approach?
Do you have any experience with it?

Dr. Rothenberg

Generally, we don't begin to do enough respite care because we
don't have enough settings in which to provide it. The unavailability of extended care facilities for children in this country is
another example of a national conspiracy against children which I
happen to have strong feelings about. Even if you do have a respite
facility available, you have to be extremely careful about approaching a family on an individual basis in terms of their need for it.
Stan's family gives a very good example of this point. If they
interpreted your offer of respite care as a criticism of their
ability to go on caring for Stan, they would find it very difficult
to accept such an offer. On the other hand, if you have a supportive
and mutually trusting relationship with a family, then they can
comfortably accept a brief period of respite care, even if it is
just for a weekend.

Dr. Dorothy Ramsey

I am thinking about an acute care setting.

Dr. Rothenberg

Yes! I agree with the "social admit or respite care admit"
to an acute pediatric setting. In this way, the other family

members can go off and catch up on sleep, or the parents can have
a weekend by themselves and not have to be worried that some terrible
medical emergency is going to be unmet.

Mrs. Christ

Could you comment on the frequency with which you see the
symptom of obesity in mothers of chronically ill children, and
whether you considered more intensive individual work with this
mother?

Dr. Christ

You have seen that in your own setting?

Mrs. Christ

Yes! It is something that we haven't really looked at system-
atically, but it is certainly a very strong impression of all the
social workers at Memorial Sloan Kettering that many of the mothers
of the chronically ill children gradually gain moderate to considerable weight.

Dr. Rothenberg

I have been struck by the same thing in a whole variety of
chronic illnesses. The dynamic is pretty straightforward in terms
of people who are feeling drained and empty by the demand being
made on them, who try to fill up this empty space by eating. On
the other hand, I am not so sure about how actively I want to intervene in all of these cases. Because of the way I edited this tape,
you couldn't see the degree to which Stan's mother wholly controls
the interview. In fact, when you see the whole interview, you
observe that this father repeatedly begins to speak, and is
interrupted by his wife. The mother is not an individual who could
feel comfortable about recognizing a need in herself for any support,
and, certainly, she would see therapy as too intrusive. Frankly,
I get very pragmatic in these instances, and hesitate to intrude
unless the situation presents an acute danger to the physical health
of the parent. I feel weight gain is a modest price to pay if all
else is equal and care is being given and things are otherwise going
okay. My own clinical goals are not to try to restore the parents
to the baseline that existed before these youngsters get sick. I
don't think one could do that. Especially with fatally ill youngsters, what I am looking for is a clarification of the new baseline,
one which can provide a new homeostatic equilibrium. One needs to
be careful not to get too judgemental, and to watch out in terms
of how modest or ambitious our own goals ought to be for these
people.

Dr. Hal Strolick: Audience Member--Family Physician

I have three things I would like you to comment on: One is
the role of the extended family in this and other families; two,
the fact that Stan seems to be, at least in this part of the interview, the only family member with a name; and three, the importance
of recognizing the family's expertise on this particular kind
of illness and dealing with a medical care system which likes to
keep the expertise to itself.

Dr. Rothenberg

Those are three critical questions. If you have an ideal
extended family, which you rarely have, it can make all the difference in the world for most folks dealing with this kind of a problem.
An ideal extended family is mutually supportive to each other, and
provides the respite care that we were just talking about. Because
many extended families are geographically so far removed, you have
to use an acute hospital for respite care, which is awful in terms
of medical economics and the whole system.

You are really sharp to pick out that Stan is the only one
with a name. I can't tell you why they call each other Mama and
Papa. They have always called themselves Mama and Papa, and refer
to each other that way. They don't refer to their children by their
first names; they talk about the "oldest boy", and "the girl"
and the "younger boy." This is not a family that I knew personally
or clinically. The case presentation and the interview were preceded by an excellent thumb-nail case presentation and history by
the pediatric resident. It could be that the other doctors who
had taken care of this family had so focused on Stan, that they
had, in fact, partially depersonalized the other children. One
sees that in families with a very sick child. It could also be
the circumstances of the interview.

And, finally, a very critical point which did not come out
in the edited interview was the degree to which these parents had
in fact learned an amazing amount about Stan's illness. For example,
they could recognize patterns that were leading to status epilepticus; they could recognize when Stan would be slipping. They had
more than one experience when they would take Stan, having a seizure,
to the Emergency Room. They would get a pediatric intern or first
year resident who didn't know them. The parents would try to explain
who they were, who Stan was, that he was known to our hospital,
what was going on, and what needed to be done. Then they would get
hassled. They got a very defensive house officer, who is essentially
but nonverbally, saying "Who the hell do you think you are, telling
me how to treat your kid?" You saw one little piece of this in
the videotape when the mother giggled and said, "I like to outguess

the doctors, and I guess I really should't do it." Well it gives
her a real sense of competence and control that she, in fact, usually
can outguess the interns and most of the residents. The neurology
residents and the neurosurgeons knew more than she did, but they
were the only ones. I think we frequently fail to take advantage
of a family's developing knowledge about their child's illness,
and to use the family as you might an extended health care provider
in meaningful ways.

This gets to the whole issue of compliance which I want to talk
about tomorrow. I would like to banish that word from the medical
lexicon. To me, compliance means: "You are sick; I am well."
"You are dumb; I am smart." "You comply with me; "I'll give you
a good reward." "I will call you a good patient or a good family
if you comply with my orders. If not, you are going to be a bad
patient or a bad family."

Dr. John Sargent

I don't think we have talked about the meaning of this
experience for this family. How do they get their rewards? I
would suggest the competence that Dr. Rothenberg just described is
one way in which a family gets rewards. If we are going to be
supporting families through experiences like this one, we need to
let them know what they are doing right, and how they are doing well.

Dr. Christ

Have any of you used a network "therapy" approach, perhaps with
the extended family or, as Dr. Dorothy Gartner has in the Downstate
Child Adolescent Division, with neighbors and acquaintances where
there is no family other than the single parent?

Dr. Hess Haber: Audience Member--Nurse

I found it helpful to have a primary care provider coordinate
everyone, much like a family therapist. This requires coordination
of the medical care, the nursing care, the social work care, etc.,
for these families. That person can periodically pull in family
members and other extended care givers to answer questions and help
them through the situation.

Dr. Christ

Have you had experience in doing that?

Dr. Hess Haber

Yes.

Dr. Christ

In what ways have you found it helpful?

Dr. Hess Haber

One of the major issues with families that are in and out of
acute care facilities is funding. Who pays for this coordinator?
I have done it as a doctoral student in Pittsburgh and on a volunteer
basis because the funding for this person is lacking. In terms of
clinical effect, it's very helpful. The issue of compliance is a
perfect example. The family knows that's going on. If they can
help to coordinate what's going on and if there is continuity of
care, then there is no problem with compliance. Families want to
be involved, and they help to make the rules. When you take part
in decision making, then you are a part of the team and there's no
issue of compliance.

Dr. Christ

Thank you. Has anybody else had experience with involvement
of the extended family?

Dr. Marshall Mintz: Audience Member--Psychologist

Not so much with the extended family. I worked with an
association of parents in New Jersey who started a network amongst
themselves which really grew out of one parent who stopped waiting
for the professionals to provide her with what she needed in terms
of emotional support. What these parents did was to create an
organization for themselves. I think it is very useful to mobilize
parents, and then to say that they can do as much as we professionals
in providing a network. Parents are really willing to jump out
and take charge, once we say that we can't do it all and, too
often, I think we, as professionals, try to provide too much.

Dr. John Sargent

As a structuralist, I want to emphasize that we must recognize
hierarchy when dealing with extended families. Too often, when we
get extended families involved, there can be a tremendous amount
of contention between the parents and the grandparents about who
is going to be doing what, how is it being done, and who cares the
most, etc., etc. People need the suggestion to go to extended
family members for help, but they also need some support to do it
in a way that is effective.

Dr. Rothenberg

Dr. Patricia MacElveen is a nurse sociologist in Seattle, who

has been working for many years on the whole issue of family networks
particularly in relation to chronic renal dialysis patients. Seattle
is a major dialysis center because that's where the technique was
worked out. Dr. MacElveen works with severely disadvantaged
families like American Indian families who are as disadvantaged as
you could imagine in your wildest nightmare. She works with another
woman, who is herself a native American Indian with anthropological
training. They have been able to pay attention to the structural
issues which Dr. Sargent just pointed out. They have been successful
with severely fragmented, disadvantaged families who are under
terrible social stress and have been chronically incapacitated
psychologically even before the acute illness appeared in the family.
I find it very, very hopeful that if we can get more people aware
of the technique of family networking, we could provide a good deal
more for a lot of these families than what we are currently doing.

Dr. Welch: Audience Member--Child Psychiatrist

I have two questions. The first is a follow-up on Dr. Sargent's
comment about what happened to the mother. We know from the literature on leukemic children of the high incidence of divorce following
the death of the child. What kind of aftercare or follow-up was
provided for this family? What often happens is that after the child
dies, that sort of closes the case.

The other issue relates to the shopping around "syndrome" found
in families with a serious chronic illness whose anxiety has not been
dealt with. How do you contain family's anxiety in a medical center
where they can go from one consultant to another? Stan's family
showed the benefit of early intervention. They have a good bit of
strength, appear to be connected to the institution and to the
program, and therefore, unlikely to shop around.

Dr. Rothenberg

I can only give you a one-year follow-up. This family was
followed by one of our superb nurse clinicians during the last two
years of Stan's life, and for a year following his death. Up until
one year following his death, the family had remained intact. The
mother had turned to the next older child, Stan's brother, and to
her teenage daughter, lavishing more attention on the two of them
than she had before. She lavished so much attention on them that
we became concerned about how over-protective she was being with
them and how that might affect their future. They were then lost
to follow-up because we didn't make intensive efforts to keep
following them. Certainly, the whole issue of post-mortem follow-up
as a rational and critical part of continuity of care is one that
we simply don't pay enough attention to. If you look from one
clinical setting to another, you find that it is the exception

rather than the rule to have an organized attempt to follow these
families for any significant period of time following the death of
a child. We know that this is a critical point at which many family
disruptions occur. It's a whole unmet need.

In reference to the issue of the "shopping around family," I
think you've suggested in your question the answer to that one.
Many of our "shopping around families", barring those who really
have some intensive psychopathology, are shopping around because,
in fact, they have never had an opportunity to get the five basic
questions answered. They have never had an opportunity to ventilate
their "FAGS Syndrome" in a setting in which they would really be
supported. The way to help them stop shopping around is to sit
down with them at the first opportunity and begin to try to find out
where they are with all of these issues in a warm and supportive
way. Unhappily, this tends to be a rather bad disease, in the
sense that families who bounce from place to place too long get to
be like foster children, who have gone to too many foster homes.
Even if they arrive the fourth time around at a really good one,
their ability to relate to that setting may have been so thoroughly
destroyed that it's too late; and sometimes you see families who
have gone that far.

ISSUES AND CHALLENGES: CONCLUDING PANEL DISCUSSION

Dr. Robert Miller - Audience Member - Psychiatrist

One of the important themes that almost everybody has talked
about is information, education, and reality orientation. In
practical experience, though, one sometimes runs into families
where information is confusing, when they misinterpret it; or when
at the time, they need to make most important decisions, they
really can't make a choice on their own. The families really need
somebody to say: "This is what's indicated." Not all families,
but some. I am in full agreement with the general theme, but there
is this other side. How do you take care of these other issues?
This hasn't been addressed by the conference.

Dr. Gabriel

I was talking to Dr. Kaplan about the early efforts to clarify
the disease or disturbance, and to help the parents learn to deal
with that. This is also critical in developmental disabilities.
Frequently, we do not clarify the problems early enough for the
parents so as to give them adequate time that they can show us that
they understand their child's problem and understand what the
alternatives are. It's a time consuming process which makes it a
difficult one for many physicians to undertake.

Dr. Rothenberg

There is a lot of this kind of problem around. No matter what
system you look at, the buck has to stop with somebody. When you
deal with a failure in medical illness, the failure is at some
point with the physician. The only way to address this is through
the educational systems for physicians. Now that may not always be
true, but certainly with very serious oncological, cardiological
and severe chronic illnesses, that point is probably not ever going
to be very much different. If there is a failure, it probably is
a reflection of the medical system, and one does the best one can
under those circumstances. But I think our fragmentation, poor

systems organization, and the whole growth of the health care
factory have contributed to this failure. Unfortunately, health
care is provided like more and more of a factory and less and less
of a humanly responsive organization.

Dr. Christ

As an administrator, I've learned one principle that I feel
touches on the question raised: When I open a discussion, I have to
be very clear whether we are going to make a mutual decision or
whether I will make a decision after adequate discussion has taken
place. There are decisions that must be made by a physician, some
that must be made by a parent, some that must be made by the child,
and some that must be made by mutual agreement. The problem you
pose is where a parent decision needs to be made, but the parent
is unable to make it. In my experience, a frank discussion about
this very issue, adding a willingness to share all information that
is required to arrive at a decision, takes care of most of these
problems. Only rarely do I go a final step, and describe how and
why I would make one or another decision AS A PARENT, but clarify
that just because I am a professional, my parent decisions do not
carry the expertise that my professional decisions do.

Dr. Rothenberg

I want to second what Dr. Christ has said. Dr. Gabriel said
that we are reacting to a tradition of medical paternalism in which
the doctor made all the decisions about everything, and was convinced that he or she knew best what was good for people. There is
evidence to indicate that people don't always know what to do with
information. But that given information, a lot of people are going
to make some pretty good decisions. One has to give the family the
option of doing that, and of having the right to decide what's
good for them. In the same way, we are arguing increasingly that
the patients should be told bad news about their illnesses and
prognosis, because they are the ones who will have to decide what
they are going to do with the rest of their lives. It's really
nobody else's business to make that decision for them.

Dr. Christ

I second the suggestion that it does take time, and that there
is a working through process. Information is provided and alternatives spelled out to patients and to families. Then they have to
work it through within their own personalities and families to
decide what they want to do. This is not always so easy for the
medical staff to get in synchrony with, when staff are oriented to
making decisions at a different pace. Often, we find it's very
hard for the medical staff to adapt themselves to the amount of

time that patients and families need to work through decisions.
But that's something no one can do for patients. You can give them
a lot of help, but you can't do it for them.

Dr. Luis N. Majerian - Audience Member - Child Psychiatrist

     I want to thank the entire panel for the very practical
clinical application yielded by the different presentations. I
would like to raise a question about another chronic pediatric
illness. Infammatory bowel disease is chronic and can affect the
child and the family at any developmental age. There are times
when the children are well functioning and it is not life threatening. I wonder if any of the panel members have had some experience
when the disease necessitates surgery. This is the point when
adaptational and functional issues come into play with the youngster,
be it a latency child or an adolescent, to determine whether or not
surgery is performed.

Dr. Rothenberg

     I have had some experience in working with children and their
families who were dealing with inflammatory bowel disease. We have
a fair amount in Seattle and, of course, it does involve working
with the gastro-enterologist and surgeons as well. In my clinical
experience, the decision to operate appears to me to be a combination
of factors that derive from everybody involved in the decision. If
you have a very powerful surgeon, powerful in terms of status in
the hospital and amongst his medical colleagues, that individual
will very often essentially make the decision. If you have a very
powerful gastro-enterologist who can control the surgeon with whom
he works, then he will often be the primary individual making the
decision. If you have a very powerful family, they just may be
able to control both those physicians and have their say about when
it's going to be done. And I am not being facetious about this.
It seems to me to depend not on anybody having done any decent
research, any decent outcome studies or anything that's based on
light, but rather on heat. The guy that generates the most heat
gets to make the decision. I think that's tragic in more than one
instance, but that seems to be the way it is.

Dr. Flomenhaft

     That applies, of course, to all diseases!

Dr. Hal Strolick - Audience Member - Family Physician

     The theme of the disorganizing effect of a crisis on a family
and translating that into a label of disorganized family or disorganized system has come up during this symposium. Since the '50s

and '60s, when people started looking at disorganized families, these were often the systems that we didn't understand. With greater attention and research, a perspective was developed where the families could be understood to be organized around things which were not obviously apparent at first glance. A lot of the apparent disorganization is actually a kind of reorganization that we are just beginning to understand. We do talk about disorganized families when, in fact, we should be talking about families whose disorganization we don't yet understand. If they are a system, they all have an organization which may be in the process of reorganization. All of us in this room, including myself as a family physician, and the panel of professionals representing major academic medical centers and great institutions, need to pause and reflect that we would never recommend to a family in crisis or recently resolving a crisis to move or make major changes. Yet often, when we do encounter a problem in a family, we immediately refer them to strange and very powerful social systems and settings without providing guides and support systems, and expect the family to respond in some kind of organized way. One wonders what kind of health care system we have become to induce disorganization and reorganization in a system that doesn't provide the kind of continuity that we saw in Dr. Christ's tape which, by the way, I greatly appreciated.

Dr. Rothenberg

    I would like to respond by thanking you, and by wishing you lived in Seattle so I could ask you to be our family doctor. I am absolutely serious about that! I wish that some of our child psychiatry fellows and advanced pediatric residents had such a good understanding of what they are trying to do.

    This also relates to a question raised yesterday about how you eliminate uncertainty for these families. We have to come to a point where we can all accept the fact that you can't eliminate uncertainty in many, if not most, of these chronic life-threatening illnesses. The issue is: How do we learn to live with it better? How do we learn to help families and patients to live with the anxiety that uncertainty and constant crisis create? And, perhaps most critically, because we pay the least attention to it, how do we as caregivers better prepare ourselves by finding a way to live with our own uncertainty about our patients and their families? By and large, we do very, very poorly with that. A significant example was when I attended an international conference of experts on death and dying several years ago. We spent five days off in the woods at a retreat. It wasn't until the fifth day that the greatest single area of difficulty surfaced, to which we had not yet addressed ourselves, and about which none of the group representing ten countries and sixty people from all over the world had done anything in an organized way: developing support systems for the

caretakers. In fact, we are rotten caretakers. This is an interesting bit of a problem, because in Greek the original word was
"caregiver." By the time it got to an Anglo Saxon form and came
down to us, it was improperly switched around to caretaker. A
caretaker is somebody who takes care <u>from</u> somebody else. People
in the health professions are great "caregivers" but rotten
"caretakers," which is why we have such a hard time developing
support systems for ourselves.

Dr. Berlin

Let me disagree with the two previous speakers because in one
sense, what you are saying is essentially very simplistic. In
my experience, disorganized families are those that have been moved
out of their context of living. For example, the Appalachian family
becomes totally disorganized after a sudden move to Seattle and
finding itself in a totally new structure. In New Mexico, the
Braceros, who have come across the border from Mexico and are now
totally disorganized, are trying to find out where they are in a
very chaotic society. I find that's also true for a variety of
American Indian families who are trying to find out where they are
in this society. Our society is a disorganizing one, and unless
one recognizes that, I think one is not really facing some of the
realities.

Dr. Strolick

Can I just respond briefly? I have worked in the South Bronx
for the last five years where we have the same problem with people
who are from Jamaica, Puerto Rico and the South. I use the term
reorganized to recognize that it is a process people are going
through in adapting the new system in a new environment, trying and
experimenting with different ways of doing that are not always as
successful as everyone would like. It's easy to close off looking
at something because it's disorganized. "Disorganized", in
general, is a punitive label. My main interest is to avoid using
a punitive label and saying that these people are failures as they
try to respond to a very powerful system.

Dr. Mattsson

Dr. Rothenberg emphasized that we have to accept uncertainty
in the execution of our various professional tasks. For decades,
medical school curricula have failed in this regard. During the
traditional first two years of medical school, the student is taught
basic sciences where so many things seem so absolutely certain.
This teaching has to be supplemented by teaching our young students
that there is nothing certain about life and their later work.

Dr. Sargent
_____

In reference to the uncertainty, after meeting with about 100
families in the course of treating an illness, they would like something to do. The families need the understanding that what they
do do is what's necessary to do, and that it's not helpful to sit
and be helpless, regardless of the existential questions.

Mrs. Christ
_____

What we observe with a lot of good coping families is that
they deal with uncertainty by becoming certain. Dr. Berlin gave
a demonstration of how he helped a family to attain coping mastery
in areas other than the area he and the family worked with. It's
a powerful coping enhancing technique to identify areas for the
families to become effective in. It may mean helping them develop
some area of personality, or of current life to enhance the feeling
of competence and enhance the impetus for growth. We have our
amputees who will say, "I was a roller skater, now I am an
excellent skate boarder with one leg." Another amputee said, "I
used to play basketball, now I am a coach." This is another way
that people deal with uncertainty.

Stephanie LeFarge- Audience Member - Developmental Psychologist
_____

There has been an unusual and admirable emphasis on using the
cognitive developmental approach in working with these children.
Would someone on the panel address the question of how acute and
chronic illness affects the progress of the child through developmental stages? How is that affected by the various coping styles
the child uses?

Dr. Rothenberg
_____

A whole conference would be in order to respond adequately to
your questions. My answer would be that it affects it in every
imaginable way. There are some kids who sublimate; instead of
getting on the skateboard, they get smart as hell and they read
faster and more than everybody else. There are other youngsters
who, because of the totality of the child's illness and the
family's value system, and a million other variables, collapse
cognitively or at least can temporarily do so. I can't do justice
to the question because it literally could be a whole symposium.

Stephanie LeFarge
_____

In my experience and in researching this area, there is a
general sense among staff that these children either are special
before they become ill or become special afterwards, becoming wiser,
sharper, and more aware, etc. etc.

Dr. Rothenberg

A lot of the kids become more aware of their illness and wiser about the medical system and the medical factory as Dr. Gabriel so aptly calls it; but it's a mistake, and I think staff are using projection and displacement, or a little of both, to imagine that every kid who has had his legs cut off is now going to become a super-genius. It makes us feel better. While I have this microphone, I cannot let the rest of the panel off the hook about this uncertainty issue. I am talking about uncertainty, about when you're going to die.

Dr. Gabriel

Isn't all life uncertain?

Dr. Rothenberg

See, that's a wise crack, and I won't accept it as a wisecrack Paul (Dr. Gabriel). All of life is not as uncertain as when you get leukemia and you are in remission--that's a whole different level of uncertainty. This isn't the first time and I am sure won't be the last symposium that I have sat through for two days in which a lot of folks are talking about chronic, life-threatening illness, and nobody wants to bite the bullet. Health professionas as a group still won't, don't, and can't develop support systems for themselves. If we do that, we have to admit we are not omnipotent or omniscient.

Dr. Kaplan

I really have to say something about that. Mrs. Christ and I were just saying, as you were talking, and I don't mean that it is unique to us because I think other groups have done it, but social workers have been developing support networks for themselves for years in medical centers. We get together and we cry on each other's shoulders because we get attached to patients just like everybody else. There is no other way to avoid burnout if you don't do that. We have done this informally and formally.

Mrs. Christ

The difference is that it's not institutionalized. That's the problem or at least one of the problems.

Dr. Kaplan

I think its happening. We are beginning to form Intensive Care Unit staff groups. It's badly needed.

Mrs. Christ

People on the front lines are doing it because they have to.

Dr. Jayakar

From my personal experience, I was a pediatrician before becoming a psychiatrist, and I decided I saw too many children dying. I remember after the third month of my rotation at Memorial Sloan Kettering, I began to feel that there are no healthy children in this world. Every child dies of leukemia, and it is a very frightening thought. One of the mothers, whose child had died, had no support system developed before or after the death of her child. She used to come into the Emergency Room and sit there with the pictures of her son to show different people how he looked before the illness. I felt that I should go and talk to her to give her some support. And all she did was hold my coat and ask me, "If I was married?" I said, "Yes, I am." She asked, "Do you have any children?" I said, "No." She responded sullenly, "Don't you ever have children, they die on you." That conversation was my most horrifying experience, and I was out of Memorial the next month. Then I got into Psychiatry and, for some reason, I am back into the same thing.

Jane Bausch - Audience Member - Graduate Social Work Student

I agree with Mrs. Christ and Dr. Kaplan that social workers do seem amazingly able to make their own support system which has been very impressive at Sydney Faber Cancer Institute in Boston. Also, I agree with Dr. Rothenberg that farther up in the hierarchy it does not seem to occur easily. The pediatric-oncologists at my hospital, to my knowledge, have no sort of support system. It is very sad. We see as one of our tasks, providing the other health care professionals with some support. It's a difficult task.

Now I would like to ask Mrs. Christ about the emotional withdrawal by the parents when they act as if the child way dead before the child is even considered a terminal case: What are the implications of that on the family system and specific interventions that you have used?

Mrs. Christ

It does have an implication for the family system. It also has a depressing impact on the patient, because the parents really aren't there either physically or emotionally. Our workers spend a lot of time monitoring the medical situation, which in this day and age is very difficult, and monitoring the family to keep the family informed about the child's medical condition and emotional adjustment.

The only thing to do is to sit down with the family and begin working with them to find out what is the source of their withdrawal, and to see if you can provide some added resource. Perhaps they are overwhelmed and need something else that you or someone else can provide for them; perhaps someone can intervene in the family system. I wouldn't under-estimate the task for the family in today's medical world to keep their emotions in harness with where the patient is medically when even the doctor often doesn't quite know. The most effective intervention is to prevent the withdrawal by keeping the family attuned to the state of the child's current medical condition.

Dr. Christ

Could you add a word about the other situation, where the child is almost pronounced dead, but then actually isn't? You mentioned that this is a particularly difficult situation.

Mrs. Christ

Very often, the child is thought to be dead and then suddenly goes into remission. The parents are stuck with the rage that they are going to have to go through this whole emotional experience again. Its very difficult!

Dr. Kaplan

I want to second something that Mrs. Christ said earlier about the issue of "abandonment" for the reasons that were given by the family doctor. It's also a stigmatic word, like the "disorganized" family. We are putting the blame on somebody, rather than realizing that if you live with a seriously chronically ill child, it's depleting as all hell. And if you don't feel like getting rid of him, then there is something wrong with you. We need to look at one of the signs which set in much earlier than when the family says, "Why don't you wheel the kid into the hall. You think it will catch a cold and then die. Let's get it over with." By that time, I think it's so bad, and the detachment is so great, that the likelihood of bringing something back is very remote. But it is possible to see the early signs, and this is a terribly important thing to do. We really ought not to talk about "abandonment." It is a bad term.

Joan Barth - Audience Member - Family Therapist

A lot of what we have seen and heard has been very touching. It seems that the touching is on a metaphorical level. I didn't see any real touching of anybody physically touching in any of the video tapes. I wonder if any of the people on the panel could talk about doing some of the kind of touching, like massage.

Frequently, I teach families to give massages to the whole family with all the children involved, and to make sure that the "care-givers" get massaged or do body kinds of things like yoga or tai-chee. While we have talked a lot about bodily illness, we weren't talking about really touching bodies.

Dr. Flomenhaft

It would seem to me that there is a lot of touching of these patients.

Dr. Rothenberg

You should have seen in my tape when the little boy and I hugged. That was special because it was a programmed action that his mother had taught him to do. He gave everybody a hug. I had just met these folks for the first time and I would have felt it inappropriate to get very touchy with them, until I found out how they responded to literally being touched. The point you are bring-ing up is that there isn't enough of that. Myself, I go every week to a masseuse, who uses a combination of two different massage techniques. I really consider this part of my professional life, because it makes a significant difference to me when I am able to do it. However, I would add a word of caution. There has been an awful lot of programmed, mechanised touching stuff cropping up all over the country. You get people doing it and it seems like the right thing to do because somebody says you ought to do it. The worst thing you could do is to put your arms around a family member or child and give them a hug when you don't really feel like it. Unfortunately, there is a distressing amount of that going on. I think the question was right. Probably there could be a great deal more of physical touching, if the medical profession as a group could get less uptight about it. It would probably be very helpful, but at the same time we have to be very cautious.

Dr. Christ

I think we may need to be somewhat more specific and pre-scriptive about touching. For example, I have done a lot of work with organically brain damaged youngsters in whom I find that there are certain points in time when attention focus is tremendously aided by body contact by touching the shoulder or the face. On the other hand, a schizophrenic youngster, or one with other difficulties, touching might precipitate a negative reaction and could be disintegrative for the child. I use this to illustrate the point that clinical judgment must be exercised in decisions about physical contact of any type.

Betsy Fife - Audience Member - Clinical Specialist

I want to get back to the issue of staff stress. A lot of the stress directly affects the quality of patient care. There is inevitable conflict between nurses and physicians on the unit level where decisions are being made about difficult treatment situations for patients. Everybody is tired and tense, and we haven't found a good way to handle physicians who have a really difficult time sitting down and talking about that. Our groups will include social workers, child-life workers, nurses and teachers, but the physicians are noticeably absent. Do you have any good suggestions on how to deal with that?

Dr. Christ

Yes I have one. It is only half facetious. One of the things that one has to keep in mind is that people sometimes support each other in very strange ways. I think you will find that in large institutions, physicians support each other by competing. And that what on the surface might appear as alienating, might actually be supporting.

Betsy Fife

That might meet the physician's needs, but doesn't take care of the problem that results in giving patient care. The conflict between the nurses and physicians, particularly, affects the kind of care that the patients are getting. It may be true that that helps the physicians.

Dr. Sargent

That is absolutely true. I work with the I.C.U. staff in a very large hospital. What I found is that help for the nursing staff is one thing, but what's helpful for the physicians is an entirely different type of experience. For the physicians, it's more oriented around learning and talking about cases. If you spend an hour and twenty minutes, it's the last 20 minutes twice a week that they start to talk about how they went home and lifted weights for 45 minutes the night before, even though it was 3:00 o'clock in the morning. What I try to do is to let each group know that the other group is responding to the same thing, and maybe, then they can feel some sense of uniformity.

Dr. Rothenberg

In our hospital in Seattle, the Director of Nursing and the Chief of Staff, after 10 years of effort, appointed nurses and physicians to an interaction committee. The committee, which

has been meeting now for several months, is to try to improve the
quality of interaction between our attending physicians and nursing
staff throughout the hospital. What was done was to choose key
attending physicians, who not only do a lot of business with us
but are powerful figures in the pediatric community. They are
seen as role models by a lot of other attendings and who, therefore,
if they change their behavior would get a lot of other people to
change theirs. A lot of clout coming right from the top of the
hospital has been associated with the committee. Even though they
have to meet at 7:30 in the morning, it is supposed to be prestigious
to be on it. So far, the committee has actually achieved something.
Our nurses just put on an Attending Physician's Week in which they
had posters all over the place, and they prepared special batches
of cookies. As always, the nurses, of course, are the ones who
reach out, and if you want to comment on that you won't get any
argument from me. It's a sad fact of life. The nurses even got
buttons made up, and every attending who appeared in the hospital
all last week, had a big yellow button which had printed on it,
"I am an attending. Talk to me," and the nurses all had big yellow
buttons that said "I am a nurse. I talk to Attendings." By
actual observations, the level of communication, if not the quality
but certainly the quantity of communication clearly increased last
week. When I get back to Seattle on Monday, I'll know whether we
are going to have any substantive results. First of all, you all
have to agree that it is a problem and then try to find some
problem solving approaches. In a lot of places, people don't even
reach that first level.

Audience Member

We seem to be skirting around the issue of sexism and male-
female relationships. In many ways, it reflects something about
mother being involved with the physician about the care of the
child, and the father being away at business. It's mirroring to
some degree the kind of thing that we are seeing in some of the
families.

Judith Riley - Audience Member - Social Worker

I want to get back to the touching point for just a moment.
In terms of our institutional architecture as well as daily patient
care routine, we can give families a chance to do the kind of
touching they do in their own homes--whether it's bathing, or
for adults to be alone together. During the blizzard of '78,
everyone was snowed in and our hospital had a couple of wonderful
sofa beds where several of the couples were able to spend several
nights together in a double bed for the first time in months. I
think that is something we might pay attention to in the future.

Dr. Flomenhaft

It's on that note that we have to close. I want to thank
all of you for a most exciting two days I have ever spent. I
thank the panel and the audience.

This final discussion highlighted a key issue of the symposium:
How to deal with "uncertainty" in treating children who have chronic,
life-threatening diseases for which there are no cures? Notwith-
standing this uncertainty, treatment decisions must be made which
have to reconcile the needs of the patient, family, and caregivers. Clearly, parents require adequate information and time in
order to understand their child's problem and consider the realistic
alternatives. One presenter noted that we must move away from a
medical paternalism and provide more opportunity for families to
participate in the decision-making process in a more humane and
responsive way. Medical staffs may have difficulty with this
process because it may mean abrogating final decision-making
responsibility and authority, and families not only take a much
longer time to work through their decisions, but ultimately may make
decisions that are contrary to the medical staff's recommendations.

The panelists agreed generally that involvement with children
who have life-threatening illnesses creates overwhelming stress for
families and caregivers. As a rule, families cope with this stress
by instinctively turning to each other for support. Contrastingly,
physicians do a very poor job of providing support for each other,
whereas nurses and social workers are more likely to give each other
support. The estrangement of the physician from this group process
can cause considerable conflict on the unit level in the care of
the patient.

In summary, this symposium highlighted the physical and psychological factors encountered by caregivers and families in understanding and treating a number of chronic and life-threatening
pediatric medical illnesses. One issue that permeated throughout
the symposium proceedings was the absence of certainty in predicting
the timing of exacerbations of death in many of the illnesses.
Nevertheless, time and time again, the panelists and audience were
reminded that both families and caregivers tended to evade this
issue. This was especially the case with the childhood and
adolescent cancer patients.

Difficult though the life experiences of these children and
families are, their struggles with their realities, as described
by the presenters, are not only enlightening, but inspiring and
moving.

CONTRIBUTORS

Irving N. Berlin, M.D.   Professor of Psychiatry and Pediatrics
                             University of New Mexico
                             School of Medicine
                             Albuquerque, New Mexico

Grace Christ, M.S.W.   Director, Social Services
                             Memorial Sloan-Kettering Cancer Center
                             New York, New York

Adolph E. Christ, M.D.   Associate Professor
                             Director, Division of Child and Adolescent
                             Psychiatry
                             Downstate Medical Center
                             Kings County Hospital Center
                             Brooklyn, New York

Delores Danilowicz, M.D.   Associate Professor of Pediatrics
                             New York University Medical Center
                             New York, New York

Peter Dunn, M.D.   Clinical Assistant Professor
                             Director of Family Therapy
                             Department of Psychiatry
                             Downstate Medical Center
                             Kings County Hospital Center
                             Brooklyn, New York

Kalman Flomenhaft, Ph.D.   Clinical Associate Professor
                             Director of Family Therapy
                             Division of Child and Adolescent
                             Psychiatry
                             Downstate Medical Center
                             Kings County Hospital Center
                             Brooklyn, New York

Hugh Paul Gabriel, M.D.   Associate Professor of Psychiatry
                             New York University Medical Center
                             New York, New York

205

Kushalata Jayakar, M.D.   Clinical Instructor
                                 Director
                                 Brooklyn Family Center/Pediatric Liaison
                                 Division of Child and Adolescent
                                 Psychiatry
                                 Downstate Medical Center
                                 Kings County Hospital Center
                                 Brooklyn, New York

David M. Kaplan, Ph.D.   Professor of Clinical Social Work
                                 Department of Family and Community Medicine
                                 Stanford School of Medicine
                                 Stanford University Medical Center
                                 Stanford, California

Åke Mattsson, M.D.   Professor of Psychiatry and Pediatrics
                                 Director, Division of Child and
                                 Adolescent Psychiatry
                                 New York University Medical Center
                                 New York, New York

Michael B. Rothenberg, M.D.   Professor of Psychiatry and Pediatrics
                                 University of Washington
                                 School of Medicine
                                 Head, Pediatric Liaison Division
                                 Department of Behavioral Sciences
                                 Children's Orthopedic Hospital and
                                 Medical Center
                                 Seattle, Washington

John Sargent, M.D.   Staff Psychiatrist and Pediatrician
                                 Philadelphia Child Guidance Clinic
                                 Philadelphia, Pennsylvania

INDEX